General Veterinary Microbiology

— An Introduction —

The Authors

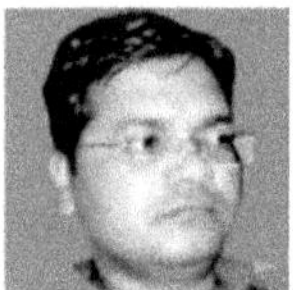

Dr. R. P. Diwakar earned his master's degree in Veterinary Microbiology from the College of Veterinary Science and Animal Husbandry, NDUA and T, Kumarganj, Faizabad. Presently, Dr. Diwakar is working as an Assistant Professor, Department of Veterinary Microbiology, College of Veterinary Science and Animal Husbandry, N.D.U. & T. Kumarganj, Faizabad (U.P). He served as Teaching Associate in Department of Veterinary Microbiology of the same University. Dr. Diwakar worked as Veterinary Officer in the State Government and as SRF in research unit, Institute of Biotechnology, Patwadagar, Nainital (U.K). He qualified ICAR-NET and published more than 22 research articles/review articles/short communication/popular articles in different national and international journals of repute.

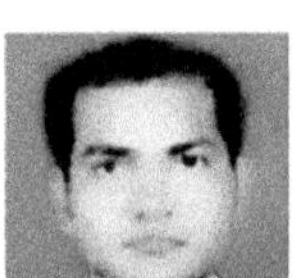

Dr. R. K. Diwakar obtained master's degree in Veterinary Public Health and Epidemiology from the College of Veterinary Science and Animal Husbandry, NDUA and T, Kumarganj, Faizabad (U.P). He has been awarded a gold medal in M.V.Sc. degree and qualified ICAR-NET. He worked as Teaching Associate in College of Veterinary Science and Animal Husbandry, Bharatpur (Rajasthan). He has published more than 07 research/review articles in national and international journals of repute. Presently, Dr. Diwakar is working as a Veterinary Officer, Department of Animal Husbandry, Govt. of Uttar Pradesh.

General Veterinary Microbiology

— An Introduction —

(As per VCI Syllabus for B.V.Sc and A.H. Degree Programme)

– Authors –

R.P. Diwakar

Assistant Professor,
Department of Veterinary Microbiology,
Narendra Deva University of Agriculture and Technology,
Faizabad (Uttar Pradesh) – 224229

R.K.Diwakar

Veterinary Medical Officer,
Department of Animal Husbandry,
Uttar Pradesh Government

2018

Daya Publishing House®

A Division of

Astral International Pvt. Ltd.

New Delhi – 110 002

Publisher's Note:

Every possible effort has been made to ensure that the information contained in this book is accurate at the time of going to press, and the publisher and author cannot accept responsibility for any errors or omissions, however caused. No responsibility for loss or damage occasioned to any person acting, or refraining from action, as a result of the material in this publication can be accepted by the editor, the publisher or the author. The Publisher is not associated with any product or vendor mentioned in the book. The contents of this work are intended to further general scientific research, understanding and discussion only. Readers should consult with a specialist where appropriate.

Every effort has been made to trace the owners of copyright material used in this book, if any. The author and the publisher will be grateful for any omission brought to their notice for acknowledgement in the future editions of the book.

Cataloging in Publication Data--DK
Courtesy: D.K. Agencies (P) Ltd. <docinfo@dkagencies.com>

Diwakar, R. P., author.
General veterinary microbiology : an introduction : as per VCI syllabus for B.V.Sc and A.H. degree programme / authors, R.P. Diwakar, R.K. Diwakar.
pages cm
Includes index.
ISBN 9789387057326 (International Edition)

1. Veterinary microbiology. I. Diwakar, R. K., author. II. Title.

LCC SF780.2.D59 2018 | DDC 636.089601 23

Published by : **Daya Publishing House®**
A Division of
Astral International Pvt. Ltd.
– ISO 9001:2015 Certified Company –
4736/23, Ansari Road, Darya Ganj
New Delhi-110 002
Ph. 011-43549197, 23278134
E-mail: info@astralint.com
Website: www.astralint.com

Dedicated to Beloved

— Parents —

Acknowledgements

We wish to put on record our sincere thanks to Dr. R.K Joshi, Professor and Head, Department of Veterinary Microbiology, Dr. D. Niyogi, Associate Professor and Head Department of Veterinary Pathology and Dr. A.K. Gangwar, Associate Professor, Department of Veterinary Surgery and Radiology and Dr. Vibha Yadav, Assistant Professor, Department of Veterinary Microbiology for making valuable suggestion during preparation of manuscript.

We wish to express our heartfelt gratefulness to Dr. Namita Joshi, Professor and Head, Department of Veterinary Pathology and Epidemiology, Dr. H. N. Singh, Dean College of Veterinary Science and Animal Husbandry for their valuable suggestion, constant encouragement.

The completion of this textbook would not have been possible without the continuous support of our family's members.

I express my indebtedness to my mother Smt. Savitri Devi and my wife Neelam Singh who had always been a constant source of inspiration, encouragement, and cooperate and help during the preparation of this book.

R.P. Diwakar

Finally, I extend my acknowledgements with gratitude, the support and love of my family- my mother Smt Savitri devi and my wife Deepti. They all help me for preparation of this book.

R.K. Diwakar

Preface

We have written this textbook with the hope to provide useful as well as informative to the undergraduate veterinary students according to Veterinary Council of India syllabus (New VCI syllabus). General Veterinary Microbiology is one of the major areas of studies in Veterinary Sciences.

This book has been prepared as per the VCI syllabus for B.V.Sc and A.H., degree programme and is divided into four parts in which practical aspect is also cover so that students easily understand and applied in field after completing the degree programmed and ultimately farmers are benefited.

Overall this book covers the general aspect of bacteria, fungi and viruses. How these are survive in nature. How resistant developed against antimicrobial agent etc which is necessary to a vetenarians or a students.

R.P. Diwakar

R.K. Diwakar

Contents

PART 2

PART 3

PART 4

Abbreviations

BEK = Bovine embryonic Kidney
BVD = Bovine virus diarrhea
CEF = Chick embryo fibroblast
CPE = Cytopathic effect
ds = Double standard
Epith = Epithelium
FBS = Fetal bovine serum
Fib = Fibroblast like
FMDV = Foot and mouth disease virus
HEL = Human embryonic lung
HSV = Herpes simplex virus
MEF = Mouse embryonic Kidney
PI3 = Parainfluenza3
RS = Respiratory syncytial
ss = Single stranded
SV_{40} = Siminian virus 40
TSI = Triple Sugar Iron
VP = Voges – Proskauer
VSR = Vesicular Stomatitis Virus

Part 1

Chapter 1

Introduction and History of Microbiology

Introduction

Through the strenous efforts put in by the fore runners of microbiology, we are at the fortunate level of knowledge now. But we often do not remembers the back ground circumstances in which the tools of investigations evolved, with this, we run the risk of getting reduced to the status of mechanical scientist instead of tract of a dynamic and vibrant one. Genesis of microbiological tools has a very long history and it may be interesting to recall that some of the tools originated at a time when microbiology itself had not distinguished itself from general biology. In this back ground, effort has been made to unearth the information on microbiology and microbiological tools and place them in proper historical perspective.

History

In the early stage of the development of science, physicians and Hippocrates (460-375 BC), Verona (2nd century, BC), Galen (130-200A.D.) and many other great scientist of that time the living nature of contagious disease was stated. At the beginning of the 17th century due to the success attained in the field of optics the previously unknown invisible mysterious world of microorganisms was discovered.

In 1590, Hans and Zaccharivs was constracted a device with magnifying lens which permitted to see minute specimens.

In microbiology field first time, Galileo Galilei (1609-1610) made first simple microscope as time passes in year 1617-1619, C. Drebbel invented the double lenses microscope with single convex objective Antony Van Leeuwenhook (1632-1723) first observed and described microbes under microscope.

The development of microbiology as a scientific disciple date from Lovis Pasteur (1822-95), a French scientist, chemist and microbiologist, his studies on fermentation. He established that fermentation was the result of microbial activity associated with different types of microorganisms (1857). The basic principles and techniques of microbiology were evolved by Pasteur. He introduced different techniques of sterilization and developed steam sterilizer, hot air oven and autoclave, he also established the differing growth needs for different bacteria his work solve major problems not only in France but entire world in various fields. Pasteur investigated the causative agents of anthrax, chicken cholera and hydrophobia. An accidental observation that chicken cholera bacillus cultures left on the bench for several weeks lost their pathogenic property but retained their ability to protect the birds against subsequent infection by them led to the discovery of the process of attenuation and the development of live vaccines. It was Pasteur who coined the term vaccine for such prophylactic preparations to commemorate the first of such preparations, namely cow pox, employed by Jenner for protection against small pox. The greatest impact in medicine was made by Pasteure's development of a vaccine for hydrophobia. This was acclaimed throughout the world.

The advancement in bacteriology took place with the improved method of investigations of Robert Koch (1843-1910), the German scientist. He has developed the experimental methodology that proved a casual relationship between bacteria and infectious disease.

In 1928, Griffith described the permanent transformation of *pneumococcus* and in 1944. Avery and his colleagues further advance the knowledge in bacterial genetics. In 1952, Zinder and Lederberg found that bacteriophages when infect bacteria can carry part of the bacterial chromosome with them when they leave one bacterium and infect another. Further important discoveries in bacterial genetics took place during middle of the twentieth century. The development in understanding the biochemical mechanism of heredity and bacterical variation and development of molecular biology.

Name of Great Microbiologist and their Contribution

Year	*Name of Microbiologist Scientist*	*Contribution*
1860	Ignaz Semmelweis Country – Hungarian	Developed statistical analysis that demonstrated that rigorous hand-washing technique.
36BC	Marcus Terentius Varro Country – Roman	Earliest proposal of the germ theory.
1884	Hans Christian Gram Country – Denmark	Developed the gram staining technique that is used to identify and classify bacteria.
1880	Charles Lavaran Country – France	Discovered malaria is caused by a protozoan.
1765	Lazzaro Spallanzani Country – Italian	Proved that bacteria did not arise due to spontaneous generation by developing the sealed, sterile broth medium.
1861	Louis Pasteur V French	Developed the germ theory of disease

Year	Name of Microbiologist Scientist	Contribution
1884	Fanny Hesse Country – German	Discovered the use of agar in bacterial culturing.
1796	Edward Jenner Country – Engligh	Discovered and applied vaccination techniques against smallpox.
1673	Antony van Leewenhoek Country – Dutch/Holland	Developed lens grinding and the first microscope, provided the first description of animicules, protozoans, fungi and bacteria.
1901	Emil Adolf von Behring Country – Germany	The novel prize for physiology and Medicine for his work on serum therapy.
1902	Sir Ronald Ross Country – United Kingdom India	The novel prize for work on malaria.
1905	Robert Koch Country – Germany	The novel prize for his investigation and discoveries in relation to tuberculosis.
1907	Charles Louis Alphonse Country – France	The novel prize for his work to recognition of playing role of protozoa in causing disease.
1928	Charles Jules Henri Nicolle Country – France	The novel prize for his work on typhus.
1939	Gerhard Domgk Country – Germany	The novel prize for discovery of the antibacterial effects of prontosil.
	Sir Alexander Fleming Country – United Kingdom	
1945	Sir Ernst Boris Chain Country – United Kingdom	The novel prize for discovery of penicillin and its curative effect in various infectious diseases.
	Howard Walter Florey	
1952	Selman Abraham Waksman Country – United state	The novel prize for Identification of streptomycin antibiotics

Chapter 2

Classification and Nomenclature of Bacteria

The science of classification of living forms is called Taxonomy, from the Greek words for law and order.

Bacterial taxonomy comprises three components.

1. Classification or the orderly arrangement of units.
2. An unknown organism can be identified and grouped or classification with other organisms that have similar characteristics
3. Nomenclature of the naming of units, taxonomy is basic and necessary tool for scientist as it provides universal language of communication.

Phylogenetic Relationship

According to Charles Darwin. 1859, evolution theory, many similarities among organisms are a result of their descent form common ancestors; so, the arrangement of organisms into taxonomic categories (called taxas) reflects degree of relatedness among them. In other words, hierarchy of taxas shows evolutionary or phylogenetic relationships.

Prokaryotes and Eukaryotes

The term prokaryotes were introduced by Edward Chatton (1937) to distinguish cells with no nucleus from nucleated cells (eukaryotes) from plants and animals.

Table 2.1: Comparative Features of Prokaryotic and Eukaryotic Cells

Sl.No.	Prokaryotic Cells	Eukaryotic Cells	
	Characters	Eukaryotes	Prokaryotes
1.	Nucleolus	Present	Absent
2.	Chromosomes	Several	Single
3.	Nuclear membrane	Present	Absent
4.	Mitotic division	Present	Absent
5.	Mitochondria	Present	Absent
6.	Lysosome	Present	Absent
7.	Golgi apparatus	Present	Absent
8.	Endoplasmic reticulum (ER)	Present	Absent
9.	Muramic acid	Absent	Present

A. Five-Kingdom System

Robert H. Whittaker, in 1969 proposed a five-kingdom system of biological classification, which considers prokaryotes to be ancestors of all eukaryotes. Kingdoms defined by him were named Monera, Protista, Fungi, Plantae and Animalia.

1. Kingdom prokarotae or monera

In this, include all prokaryotes.

2. Kingdom Protista

Eukaryotic organisms, mostly unicellular (and if multicellular, lacking in tissue organization) and having flagella at some times during their life-cycle, are comes under this kingdom. It includes water molds, slime molds, protozoa and eukaryotic algae.

3. Kingdom Fungi

In this, unicellular yeasts, multicellular molds and mushrooms includes. A fungus with the help of plasma-membrane absorbs organic matter. The cells of multicellular fungi are joined together to form thin tubes called hyphae. The hyphae are divided into multinucleated units by cross walls that have holes so that cytoplasm can flow between the cells like units. Most of the fungi lack flagella; they develop from spores or from fragments of hyphae.

4. Kingdom Plantae

It includes some algae and all mosses, ferns, conifers and flowering plants, all of which are multicellular. Plants obtained energy with the help of photosynthesis.

5. Kingdom Animalia

It includes various worms, sponges, insects and vertebrates. They all are obtained nutrients and energy by ingesting organic matter.

Table 2.2: Characteristics of the Five Kingdoms

Characteristics	*Five Kingdoms*				
	Monera	*Protista*	*Fungi*	*Plantae*	*Animalia*
Cell type	Prokaryotic		Eukaryotic	Eukaryotic	Eukaryotic
Cell wall	Noncellulosic (Polysacchorieds + amino-acid)	Present in some cellulose	Present without	Present cellulose	Absent
Nuclear membrane	Absent	Present	Present	Present	Present
Body organization	Cellular	Cellular	Multicellular	Tissue/organ	Tissue/organ/ organ system
Mode of nutrition	Autotrophic (Chemosynthetic and photosynthetic) and Heterotrophic (Saprophytic/parasitic)	Autotrophic (photosynthetic) and Heterotrophic	Heterotrophic (Saprophytic/ parasitic)	Autotrophic (photosynthetic)	Heterotrophic (Holozoic/ saprophytic *etc.*)

Three kingdom system, Carl Woese (1978) proposed three kingdom system on the basis of modern techniques of molecular biology and biochemistry that revealed that there are two types of prokaryotic cells. The eubacteria or true bacteria and the archaea.

Nomenclature

System of Binomial Nomenclature

Every organism has two names, genus and species. Both are printed italic or underline. The genus name is always capitalized and is always a noun. The species name is written in lower case and is usually an adjective.

Rule for assigning names to newly classified bacteria and for assigning bacteria to the taxa are established by the international committee on systematic bacteriology and are published in the bacteriological code. Description of bacteria and evidence for their classification are published in international journal of systematic bacteriology, before being incorporated into a reference called Berger's manual. According to the Bacteriological code, scientific names one to be taken from Latin (a genus name can be taken from Greek) or latinized by addition of appropriate suffix. Suffizes for order and family are – ales and – aceae respectively.

Taxonomic Hierarchy

It is a group of organisms into a series of subdivisions.

- ✰ A numbers of species make up a genus.
- ✰ Related genera make up a family.
- ✰ A group of similar families constitute a order.
- ✰ A group of similar order make up a class.
- ✰ Classes make up a division/phylum
- ✰ Division makes up a kingdom.

Phylogenic Hierarchy

It means grouping of organisms according to evolution from a common ancestor. Phylogeny can be based on other types of evidence such as nucleic acid hybridization and sequencing studies.

Classification of Bacteria

According to Bergey's manual of systematic bacteriology- bacteria have been divided into four divisions (Table 2.3).

Classification of Bacteria by following criteria

1. On the Basis of Morphological Characteristics

On the basis morphological characteristics, identify the bacteria as in structure bacteria are flagellated or endospores. It tells little about phylogenetic relationships.

Table 2.3: Bacteria Classification (Bergey's Manual)

Divisions	*Description*	*Classes*
Gram positive thick cell wall	Eubacteria	✰ Non photosynthetic bacteria ✰ Anaerobic photosynthetic bacteria ✰ Cynobacteria
Gram positive thin cell wall	Eubacteria	✰ Cooci and rods ✰ Actinomycetes and other related bacteria
Wall-less bacteria	Eubacteria	✰ Mycoplasma
Unusual cell wall	Eubacteria	

Bergey's manual provides a reference for identification of bacteria in laboratory.

2. On the Basis of differential Staining

It is first step for identification of bacteria as Gram positive, or negative, acid fast bacteria *etc.*

3. On the Basis of Biochemical Tests

Selective and differential media also based on biochemical tests/reactions.

Enzymatic activity of bacteria.

4. On the Basis of Serology

Agglutination tests, ELISA, Western blot used to identified bacterial antigen in patient's serum.

5. On the Basis of Phage Typing

Phages usually caused lysis of bacteria cells they infect, they are highly specialized and infect only members of a particular species.

6. On the Basis of Nucleic Acid Composition and their Hybridization

Used for determining evolutionary relationship between bacteria.

7. Flow Cytometry

Detect the presence of bacteria by detecting the differences in electrical conductivity between the cells and its surrounding media.

Identify the bacteria without culturing.

8. Numerical Taxonomy

Evolutionary relationship between bacteria on the basis of molecular analysis.

Chapter 3

Microscopy

Introduction

Leeuwenhook's make a great simple instrument, which open the door in microbial world. It is essential tool in the microbiology laboratory. Microscope, an optical instrument consisting of a lens or combination of lens for making magnified images of very small/minute objects, that is invisible to the eye.

Microscope is the most widely used instrument to demonstrate and study the shape, size and structure of bacteria.

Microscopes are of two categories:

A. Light microscope

B. Electron microscope

A) Light Microscope

In the ordinary optical microscope, the specimen of object, borne on a glass slide is scanned by focused beam of visible light. Parts of the specimen that are optically dense, having a high refractive index or being colored with a stain, cast a potential image, like a shadow, in the beam of light, which is magnified in two stages as it passes up the microscope into the eye of the observer.

Monocular Microscopes

The monocular microscopes have a single eyepiece. The rays of light from the objective lens are directed into the eyepiece and ultimately to the eye of the observer.

Binocular Microscopes

The binocular microscope have two eye pieces and are recommended where much microscopic work has to be done by the use of both eyes so that much eye strain

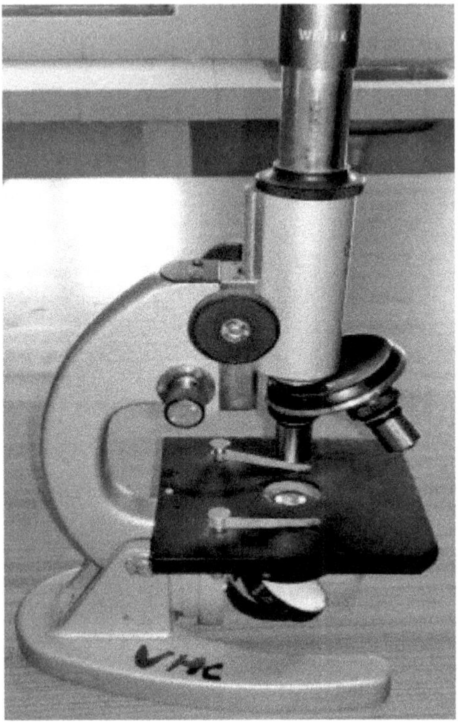

Figure 3.1: Monocular Microscope.

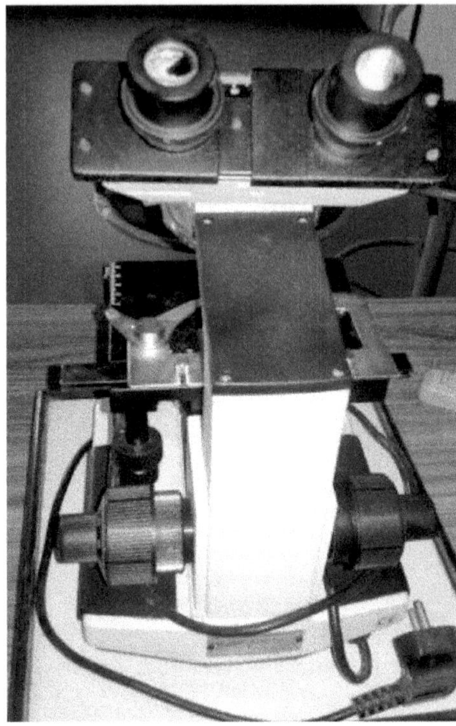

Figure 3.2: Binocular Microscope.

and fatigue is avoided. In the binocular heads, the rays of light from the objectives are divided equally by a half silvered surface inclined at 45° which permits half the light to pass through it and reflects the remainder at right angle. Each half of the rays is directed into its appropriate eyepiece by means of a prism. The inclined body may increase the overall magnification of the microscope by *e.g.* 1.5 times, when this factor will be engraved on it.

Types of Light Microscopes

1. Bright-field microscope
2. Dark- field microscope
3. Ultra-violet microscope
4. Fluorescence microscope
5. Phase contrast microscope

1. Bright-field Microscope

In this microscope, the microscopic field or area observed is brightly lightened and the object being studies appears darker. Generally microscope of this type produces a useful magnification of about 1000 diameters. However, a magnification of 1000 to 2000 diameter is the limit of useful magnification obtainable with this microscope. The microscope, which we often use in the laboratory, is called compound microscope because it has two sets of lenses; objective and ocular lens.

Resolution (or resolving power) of Microscope

It is the ability of the lenses to distinguish two adjacent points as distinct and separate. The resolving power of a microscope is depends upon the wave-length of light used and the numerical aperture (NA), which is characteristic of a lens system.

☆ Shorter the wavelength of the light used greater will be the resolution.

$$\text{Resolving power} = \frac{\text{Wave length of light (Lamda)}}{\text{NA objective + NA condenser}}$$

Wave length (Lambda) of green filter light is 0.55μm which is liked by most by the human eye.

Numerical aperture (NA) of objective is the sine valve of the half aperture angle multiplied by the refractive index 'n' of the medium filling the space between the front and the cover slip.

NA = n Sine θ

The value of 'n' is 1 with dry objectives (Since 1 is refractive index of air) while it is 1.56 when immersion oil is employed. If 0 is 58°

NA = n Sine θ (theta)

= 1.56× Sine 58°

= 1.56× 0.85

= 1.33

Thus resolving power of a microscope using oil-immersion and green light = 0.55/1.33+0.9

= 0.55/2.23

= 0.25 μm

From the calculation it is concluded that the smallest resolvable object that can be seen with the light microscope is of 0.25 μm diameter approximately. Magnification beyond the resolving power would be of no valve since larger image would be less distinct and fuzzy in appearance. The degree to which resolution from a microscope can be obtained is limited because of the limitation of wave length of visible light (0.4 to 0.7 μm) and the NA of light microscope.

Magnification

The total magnification achieved with the microscope depends on the combination of the ocular and objective lens used. There are three objective lenses on the nosepieces; low power objective lenses(10X), When an objective is viewed with 10X objective combined with 10X ocular, it is Magnified 100 time (100X). The other

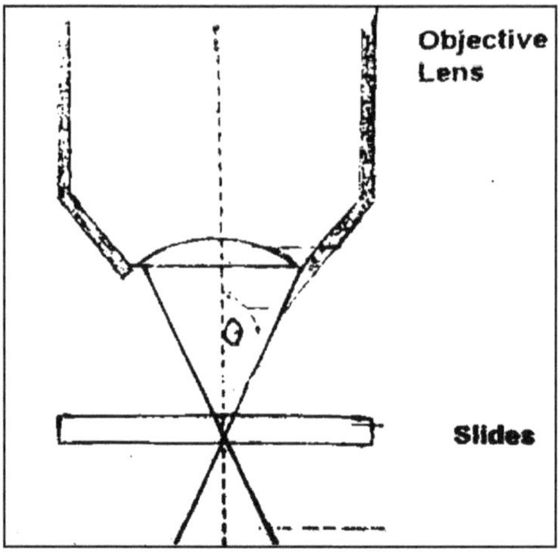

Figure 3.3: The Value of Theta is Determined as Shown in the Figure and is Needed for the Calculation of Numerical Aperture (NA).

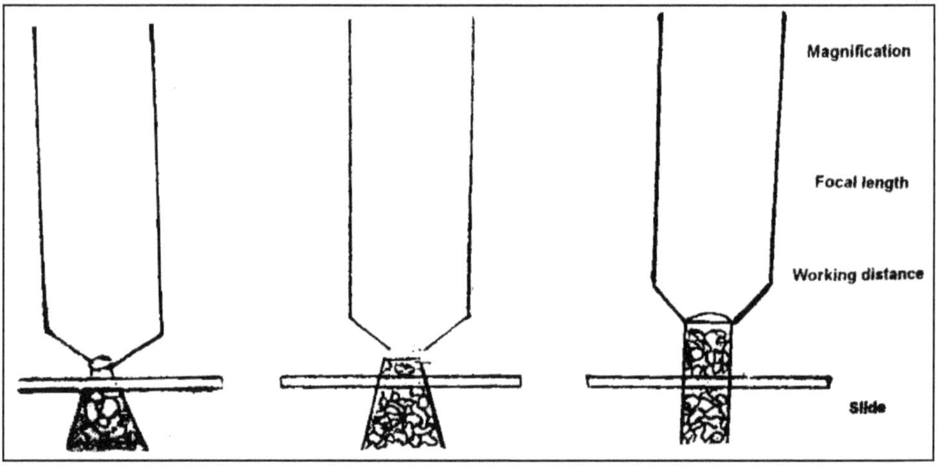

A (95×10=950) **B (44×10=440)** **C (10×10=100)**

Figure 3.4: Objective Used on a Light Microscope (A) Oil-immersion; (B) High Dry, (C) Low Power.

two objective look alike in length; high power objectives (40X) and oil-immersion objective (100X). The Oil improves the resolution of magnified image.

Why oil immersion objective lens used?

Oil-immersion objective is usually employed in the microbiological laboratory since it provides higher magnification than any other type of objective; it focuses extremely close to the specimen. The oil-immersion is required to provide an optically homogenous path for the light to travel between the slide and front lens of the objective.

As the refractive index of air is less than that of glass, many of the light rays passing through the specimen are refracted at so great an angle that they completely miss the objective. By interposing oil-immersion, which has essentially the same refractive index as glass, between the slide and the objective lens, a for greater percent of the light – rays from the specimen pass directly into the objective, resulting in greater resolution and a clear image.

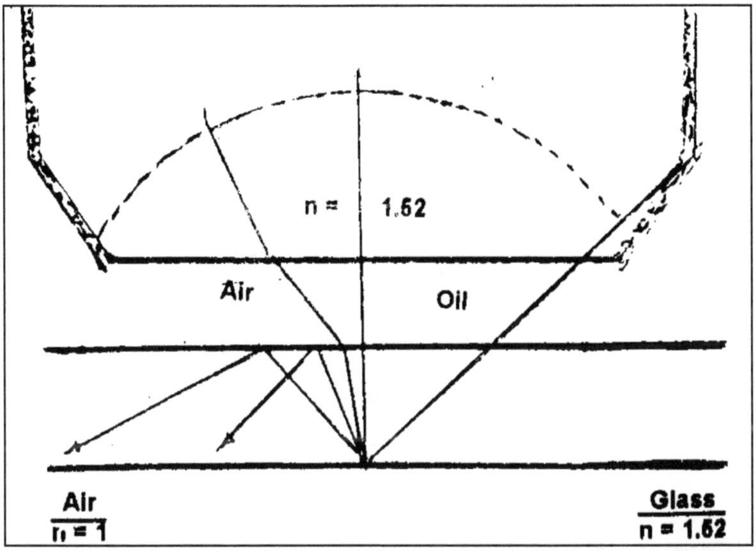

Figure 3.5: The Function of the Oil Used with the Oil-immersion Objective.

2. Dark-Field Microscope

This microscope has a dark background against which objects are brilliantly illuminated. This is accomplished by equipping the light microscope with a special kind of condenser that directs the light path from the source of illumination. Dark- field microscope is particularly valuable for the examination of **unstained microorganism** suspended in fluid 'wet' and hanging drop preparation.

3. Ultra-Violet Microscope

Ultra-violet microscope permit somewhat greater resolution, hence it produces greater useful magnification than that obtained with conventional light microscope because **Ultra-violet** light has a shorter wave length than visible light. This method is also valuable for localization, distinction and measurement of bacteria even in living state. Ultra-violet radiations are not visible; images are made visible by recording on a photographic emulsion by the use of an image converter tube or by display on a television screen.

4. Fluorescence Microscope

In this, bacteria are stained with a fluorescent dye and examined by light microscopy with Ultra-violet illumination. The stained bacteria appear luminous.

For example, fluorochrome dyes such as fluorescin isothiocynate (FITC) is used to stain Bacillus anthracis, the causative agent of anthrax, appears apple green in color.

Fluorescence microscope has been also used in diagnostic techniques such as fluorescent antibody technique (FAT).

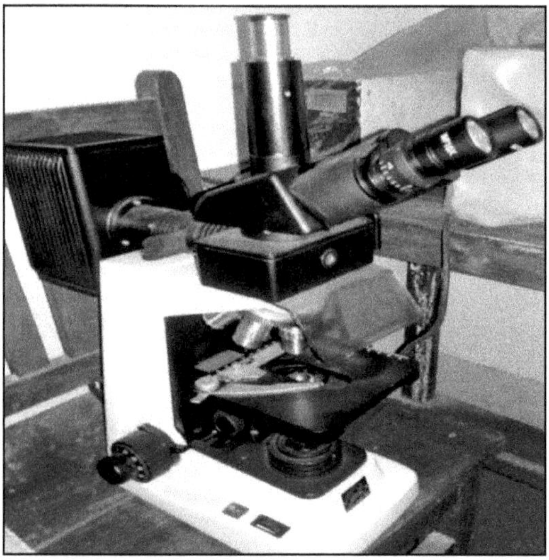

Figure 3.6: Fluorescence Microscope.

5. Phase Contrast Microscope

It is used for direct observation of unstained material. It permits the detailed investigation of the internal structure of living organism.

The principle of Phase contrast microscope is based on the slight variation in refractive index. As the rays pass from the specimen their velocity may be altered by the differences in the thickness and physical properties of various portions of the specimen. The light rays passing through the specimen are differected (bent) differently and travel at another pathways to reach the observer eye. These phase differences are seen through the microscope as the different degree of brightness. Internal structure of the specimen also become sharper and brightness against dark background.

In the **Phase contrast** microscope uses a special condenser that contain annular diaphragm. The diaphragm allows a ring of light to pass through the condenser, focusing the light on the specimen and ring shape diffraction (Phase) plate in the objective lens. The diffracted and un-diffracted rays are then brought into phase with each other to produce the image that meets the eyes.

B) Electron Microscope

Very minute objects or smaller than 0.2 µm, like viruses and internal structure can only be viewed by the electron microscope. In this microscope electron beam is used in place of light. Electrons travel in waves. The better resolution of electron microscope is due to shorter wave length of electrons. Electron microscope employed

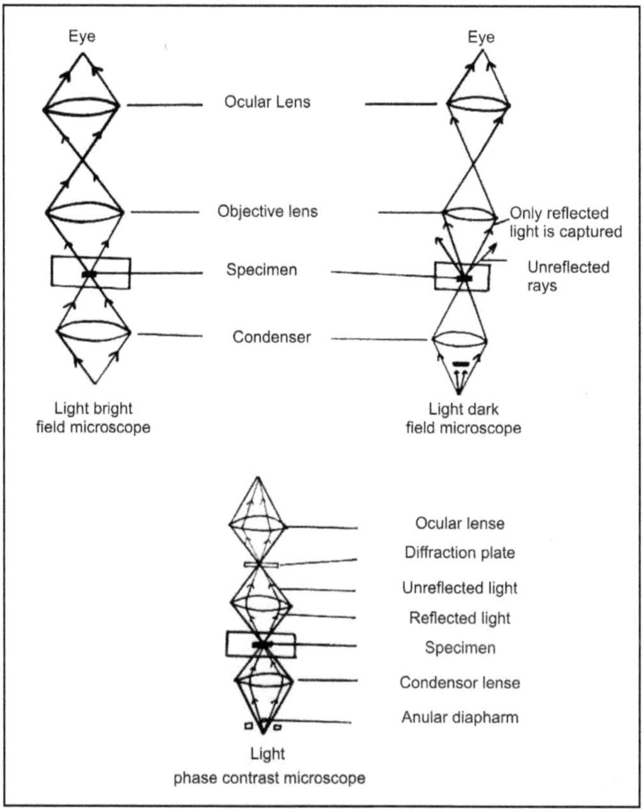

Figure 3.7: Ray – Diagrams.

60 to 80 kv electron the wave length is only 0.05A° (A° is the abbreviation for angstrom, 1 A° equals (10^{-8}) cm or 1/10,000 (10^{-4}) μm.

Electron microscope can magnify the object from 20×10^4 to 40×10^4 times its original size.

Types

1. Transmission Electron Microscopy (TEM)
2. Scanning Electron Microscopy (SEM)

1. Transmission Electron Microscopy (TEM)

In TEM, afinely focused beam of electron from an electron gun passes through a specially prepared ultra thin section of specimen.

The beam is focused on a small area of specimen by electromagnetic condenser lens. The beam of electron passes through the specimen then to the electromagnetic objective lens, which enlarge or magnifies the image. Finally, electrons are focused by electromagnetic projector lens on a fluorescent screen/photographic plate. Object can be magnified from 10,000X to 100,000X with resolution of 2.0 nm.

2. Scanning Electron Microscopy (SEM)

In SEM, electron gun produces focused beam of electron called primary electron beam. The electrons passess through electromagnetic lens and over the surface of the specimen.

The primary electrons beams knocks electron out of the surface of the specimen and secondary electron thus produced are transmitted to an electron collector amplified and are used to produce on a viewing screen SEM is used for investigation of surface structure of cells and viruses. Object can be magnified from 1000X to 10,000X with resolution of 20mm.

Chapter 4

Bacterial Structure and Morphology

Introduction

Bacteria (derived from a Greek word Bakterion means small staff) are the unicellular organisms which do not have chlorophyll and contains two types of nucleic acid, *viz.*, deoxyribo nucleic acid (DNA) and ribo nucleic acid (RNA) and also contain all the mechanisms,which is required for their growth, metabolisms and replication.

Bacteria are prokaryotic differ from Eukaryotic as discuss in **Table 2.1 (Chapter 2).**

Size of Bacteria

The size of bacteria varies from 0.1 to 16-18µ. Most of the pathogenic bacteria range from 0.2 to 5µm in length. The limit of resolution of naked eyes is about 200µ, Thus bacteria can be visualized only under a microscope. They are larger than viruses and smaller than red blood cells. *Mycoplasma* and *Rickettsias* are slightly larger than largest virus particles (*Vaccinia virus*).

Shape of Bacteria

On the basis of their shape, bacteria can be divided into four forms *viz.* spherical or cocci, rod or bacilli, spiral and filamentous.

The shape of bacteria is not constant. Bacteria may change their shape depends upon surrounding environmental condition. Bacteria are capable of retaining their specific size and shape inherited during the process of evolution. When bacteria grow under un-favorable environment, they may be found abnormal shapes. Cells of this type are called involution form or pleomorphic types. Pleamorphism of bacteria is also viewed when bacteria are grown on a artificial media.

Cocci- (Coccus - Singular)

Derived from Greek word kokkas means berry. These forms of bacteria are spherical, ellipsoidal, bean shaped and lanceolate.

Cocci are divided into six groups, on the basis of cell arrangement/cell division/ properties.

Sl.No.	*Groups*	*Structure*	*Cell Arrangement/Cell Division*
1.	Staphylococci	Staphylo= cluster of Grapes	✰ Irregular planes and arranged in clusters
2.	Streptococci	Strepto = chain	✰ Divide in one plane ✰ Arranged in chain
3.	Diplococci	Diplo = double	✰ Divide in one plane ✰ Arranged in pairs
4.	Micrococci	Single	✰ They remain singly
5.	Tetracocci	Tetra = Four	✰ Divide in two plane ✰ Arranged in group of four
6.	Sarcinae	Sarci = tie	✰ Divide in three plane ✰ Arranged in packet of eight/sixteen/more

Bacilli (Bacillus - Singular)

They are growing in single or in clusters. Bacilli are of different types, *viz.* Short or cocco bacilli, straight or long rod and Chinese letter like in appearance. Length and width are somewhat equal in case of coccobacilli and in straight bacilli the length is more compare than width.

In the rod shaped bacteria has more surface area as compare to cocci. So requirement of nutrition is more for their growth.

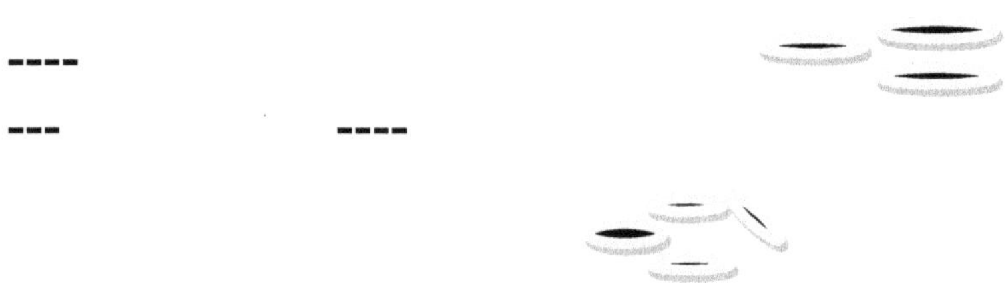

Figure 4.1: Types of Bacilli.

Spiral shaped bacteria are comma shaped, twisted, cork screw shaped and filamentous bacteria are elongated, tread like and may have branches.

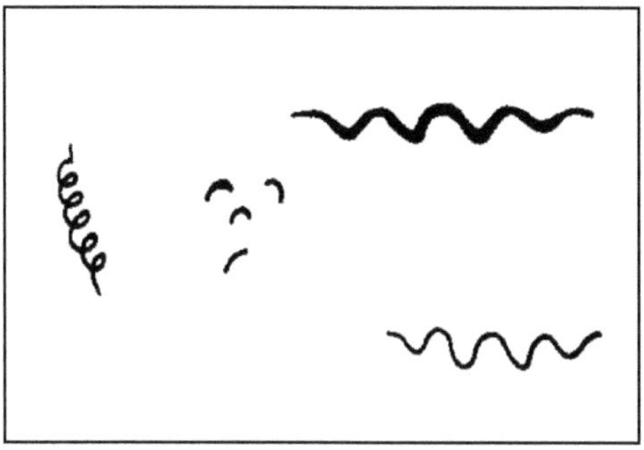

Figure 4.2: Types of Spiral Shaped Bacteria.

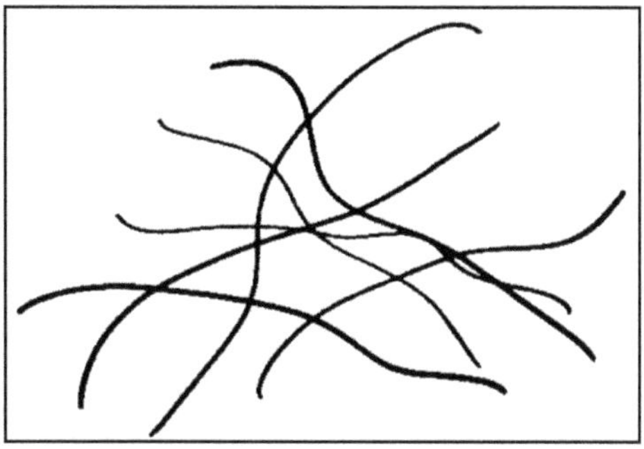

Figure 4.3: Filamentous Bacteria.

Structure of Bacterial Cells

A typical bacterial cell is containing a capsule, cell-wall, cell membrane, cytoplasm containing nuclear material and appendages like flagella and pili (fimbriae).

Some of the species of bacteria can produce forms termed spores or endospores, which are resistant to the environmental conditions.

The structural components of bacteria are seen clearly under electron microscope.

Nucleus

Bacterial nuclei can be demonstrated by acids or ribonuclease hydrolysis and subsequent staining for the nuclear material. They appear as oval or elongate bodies, generally one per cell. Some of cells possess two or more nuclear bodies due to asynchrony between nuclear and cytoplasmic division. The nucleus of a bacterium is composed of a double stranded DNA, RNA and protein at the ratio of 60:30:10.

Bacterial nuclei have no nuclear membrane or nucleolus. The nuclear deoxyribonucleic acid (DNA) is not associated with basic protein. The genome consist of a single molecules of double stranded DNA arranged in the form of a circle, which may open under certain conditions to form a long chain, about 1000μm in length. The bacterial chromosome is haploid and replicates by simple fission and by mitosis in the higher cells.

The differences between the nuclei of bacteria and higher organisms forms the main basis for classifying them as prokaryotes and eukaryotes.

Bacteria may contain extranuclear genetic elements (DNA). These cytoplasmic carriers of genetic information are termed plasmids or episomes; they may be transferred from one bacterium to another through conjugation.

Bacterial nucleus is difficult to demonstrate directly under a light microscope however discrete nuclear bodies can be recognized under a light microscope by special staining such as Robinow and Fuelgen staining method.

Cytoplasm

The bacterial cytoplasm is a colloidal mixture of (organic and inorganic solutes) water, proteins, lipids, carbohydrates, mineral compounds and other substances. It differs from eukaryotic cytoplasm.

Cytoplasm contains ribosomes, mesosomes, inclusion and vacuoles.

a) **Ribosomes** are site of protein synthesis. Groups of 50-55 ribosomes linked together and form a polysome (Smaller than the ribosome of eukaryotic cells, sedimentation constant 70S).

b) **Mesosomes (Chondroids)** are vesicular, convulated or multilaminated structures formed as an invagination of the plasma – embrane into the cytoplasm. In gram positive bacteria, they are more prominent. They play important role in cell respirationby carrying the enzymatic systems and in cell wall formation during cell-division (binary fission).

c) **Intracytoplasmic inclusion** Numerous inclusions comprising of volutin granules, polysaccharides, lipid and crystals. They are chacteristic for different species and depends upon the age and condition of the culture.

   I) **Volutin granules (metachromatic or Babes-Ernst granules)** are highly refractive, basophilic bodies consisting of poly metaphosphate.These granules are considered to be reservoir of energy and phosphate for cell metabolism. They appear reddish when stained with polychrome methylene blue or toluidine blue. By special staining techniques, such as albert or neisser demonstrate the granules more clearly.

   II) **Lipoprotein bodies-** These bodies appear as fat droplets when bacteria are grown on nutrient media of high carbohydrate content and disappear when cells are deprived of nutrients. They can be demonstrated by Sudan or fuchsin strain

   III) **Glycogen granules-** These granules can be identified when stain the cells with lugol's iodine. These granules are the reservoir of source of energy.

The bacterial cytoplasm contains vacuoles, which is fluid containing cavities separated from the cytoplasm by a membrane. Their function and significance are unclear.

Cell (Cytoplasmic) Membrane

Cytoplasmic membrane is a thin layer (5 to 10 nm) structure lies inside the cell wall and enclosing the cytoplasm of the cell. It is a complex, highly organized and specialized structure and semi-permeable in nature. Chemically Cytoplasmic membrane consists of lipoprotein with small amount of carbohydrate. Sterol is absent in Mycoplasma.

The main ones of these:

- ✰ Permeability barrier
- ✰ Electron transport and chemosomosis
- ✰ ATPase, ATP synthetase activity
- ✰ Transport of nutrients and ions
- ✰ Synthesis and transport of peptidoglycon precursors, polysaccharides, lipopolysaccharides, secreted protein
- ✰ Site of anchorage of flagella, site of rotor energization
- ✰ Chemoreceptors for chemotaxis
- ✰ Anchorage of fimbriae and pili
- ✰ Attachment point for replicating DNA

The Cell Wall

Cell wall of bacteria is a complex semi-rigid structure responsible for maintain the shape and size of bacteria. The cell wall cannot be seen by direct light microscope and does not stain with simple stains. It may be demonstrated by plasmolysis, when placed in the hyper tonic solution. Bacteria cell wall are about 10 to 25 nm thickness and account for about 20-30 per cent of dry weight of the cells.

The bacterial cell wall is composed of macromolecular network called peptidoglycon (Also known as murein), which is present either alone or with combination of the other susbstances. Peptidoglycon consist of repeating dissacharide attached by polypeptide to form a lattice that surrounds and protect the entire cell. The disaccharide portion is made up of monosaccharides called N acetylglucosamine (NAG) and N acetyl muramic acid (NAM) alternating in chains, which are cross-linked by peptide chains. The various components of peptidoglycon are assembled in the cell wall. Alternating NAG and NAM molicules are linked in rows of 10-65 sugars to form carbohydrate back bone.(glycon portion of peptidoglycan) adjacent rows are linked by polypeptide (the peptide portion of peptidoglycon). Although the structure of the polypeptides link varies. It always includes tetrapeptide side chain, which consist of four amino acid attached to NAMs in back bone. The amino acid occurs in alternating pattern of D and L forms. This is unique because the amino-acid found in other protein are L-forms. Parallel tetrapeptide side chain may be directly bounded to each other or linked by a peptide cross bridge consisting short chain of amino-acid.

Penicillin interferes with the final linking of the peptidoglycon rows by cross-bridges. As a result the cell wall is greatly weakened and the cell under goes lysis, destruction caused by rupture of the plasma-membrane and the loss of cytoplasm.

Gram Positive Cell Wall

Cell wall consist of many layers of peptidoglycon forming a thick, rigid structure (gram negative cell wall consist of thin layer of peptidoglycon), this is one reason that gram positive bacteria are more susceptible to penicillin than gram negative bacteria.

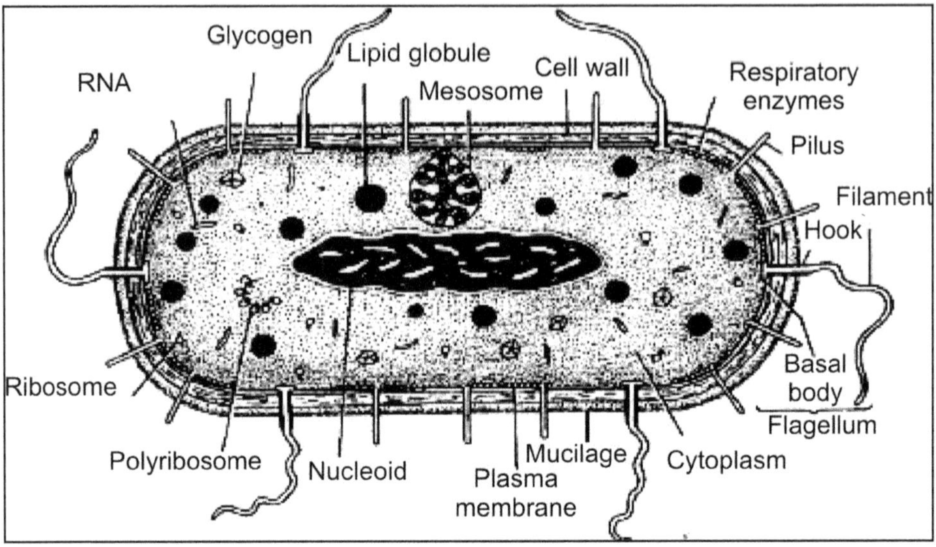

Figure 4.4: Diagram of Bacterial Cell.

Cell wall of gram positive bacteria contain teichoic acid, which consist primarily of an alcohol (glycerol/rabitol) and phosphate. There are two classess of teichoic acid.

I) **Lipo-teichoic acid -** Which spans the peptidoglycon layer and linked to the plasma-membrane.

II) **Wall-teichoic acid -** Which is linked to the peptidoglycon layer because of their negatively charge. Teichoic acid may bind and regulate the movement of cations into and out of cell.

Role of Teichoic Acid

- In the cell growth
- Preventing extensive wall break down
- Cell lysis

Teichoic acid provides much of the wall's antigenic specificity and thus make it possible to identify the bacteria.

Gram Negative Cell Wall

Cell wall of gram negative bacteria consist of one or very few layers of peptidoglycon and an outer membrane. The peptidoglycon is bounded to lipoprotein in the outer membrane and is in the periplasmic space. Periplasmic space is a space between outer membrane and plasma membrane,the periplasmic space contains a high concentration of degradative enzyme and transport proteins. Gram negative cell wall do not contain teichoic acid because cell wall of grame negative bacteria contain only a small amount of peptidoglycon and they are more susceptible to mechanical breakage.

Outer membrane of gram negative bacteria consist of lipoprotein (Lipopolysaccharides (LPS) and phospholipid).

Special Function of Outer Membrane

- ☆ Its strong negatively charges is an important factor in evading phagocytosis and the action of complement.
- ☆ Also provide a barrier to certain antibiotics, digestive enzymes like lysozyme, detergents, heavy metal, bile salt and certain dyes.

Outer membrane does not provide a barrier to all the substances in the environment because nutrient must passess through to sustain the metabolism of the cell. Permeability of the outer membrane is due to protein in the membrane called porin protein. This protein farm a channel and permit the passages of molecules such as nucleotide, disaccharides, peptides, Amino-acid, Vitamin B12 and iron. They can also make bacteria vulnerable to attack by providing attachment site for viruses and other harmful substances. The LPS component of the outer membrane (OM) provides two important characters of gram negative bacteria.

I) Polysaccharides portion is composed of sugar called 'O' polysaccharides that function as antigens and are useful for distinguishing species of gram negative bacteria.

II) Lipid portion of the LPS called Lipid A, is referred to as endotoxic activities and is toxic when the host's blood stream or GIT. It causes fever and shock.

Table 4.1: Summary of Major Structures of Bacteria, their Chemical Composition and Function

Structures	*Chemical Composition*	*Function*
Cytoplasmic membrane	Lipid and protein	☆ To control the metabolic and waste product into and out of the bacterial cells ☆ Storage of the enzymes for synthesis of protein, toxins, enzymes, nucleic acids and other substances.
Cell-wall Gram positive bacteria	Peptidoglycan, polysaccharides and teichoic acid	☆ Protect the bacterial cell ☆ Provide the shape. ☆ Take part in cell growth and cell division
Gram negative bacteria	Peptidoglycan, lipopolysaccharides, protein and lipid	
Capsules	Glycoprotein, polysaccharides and polypeptide	☆ Anti-phagocytic activity
Flagella	Protein (Flagellin)	☆ Provide motility to bacteria
Pili	Protein (Pilin)	☆ Transfer of genetic material ☆ Associated with antigenicity

Table 4.2: Comparison of Gram Positive and Gram Negative Cell Wall

Characteristic	*Gram Positive*	*Gram Negative*
Peptidoglycan	Thich 50 per cent	Thin 15-20 per cent
Terapeptide	Most have lysine	All have diaminopimelate
Cross-linkage	Generally thru pentapeptide	
Teichoic acid	Present	Absent
Lipoproteins	Absent (0 to 3 per cent)	Present (58 per cent)
Lipopolysaccahride	Absent (0 per cent)	Present (13 per cent)
Outer membrane	Absent	Present
Periplasmic space	Absent	Present
Polysaccharide	Present	Present
Protein	Present or absent	Present
Hexosamine content in cell wall	More	Less
Magnesium content	Greater	Less
Apparent isoelectric point by staining	pH2-3	pH4-5
Toxins production	Exotoxin	Endotoxin
Resistance to physical disruption	High	Low
Flagellar structure	2 ring in basal body	4 rings in basal body
Inhibition by basic dyes	High	Low
Susceptibility to anionic detergents	High	Low
Resistance to sodium azide	High	Low
Resistance to drying	High	Low
Sensitivity to penicillin G	Yes	No
Sensitivity to lysozyme	Yes	No

Morphological Variations

I) Protoplasts and Spheroplasts

Protoplasts and spheroplasts are altered form of bacteria or yeast, in which the principal shape maintaining structure of the bacteria is weakened. Each bacterium forms a sphere, which is the shape that allows the bacterium to withstand the rigors, particularly osmotic, off the fluid in which it resides.

The term protoplasts refers to the spherical shape assumed by gram positive bacteria, bacteria spheroplasts spherical shape assumed by gram negative bacteria. The difference is essentially the presence of single membrane in the case of protoplast and two membranes (inner and outer) of gram negative spheroplasts. It is also possible to generate a gram negative protoplast by the removal of outer membrane. Thus protoplast refers to a bacterial sphere that is bounded by a single membrane and spheroplasts it refers to sphere that is bounded by two membranes.

II) L-forms of Bacteria

These are protoplast and appear as a large spherical shaped and thread like plasmatic structures. The L - form has been named after the Lister institute where this form of bacteria was first discovered in 1935.

Capsule/Glycocalyx

Many bacteria synthesize and secret polysaccharide polymers around the cell surface and effectively cover it. When this is organized into a sharply defined structure, as in the *Pneumococcus*, it is known as Capsule.

It's chemical composition varied widely with the species for most part it is made inside the cell and excreted to cell surface. Generally when the smear is un-organized and only loosely attach to cell wall, the glycocalyx is called as Slime layer. When the substance is organized and is farmelly attached to cell wall, the glycocalyx is called as capsule. Capsule is a important in contributed to bacterial live. It protect to pathogenic bacteria from phagocytosis (anti-phagocytic activity) and increase the chances of colonization of bacteria by lowering the charge on the cell surface. Capsule is made up of sugar is called Extracellular polysaccharide (EPS), which enable the bacteria to attach the various surfaces. By allowing there adherence and colonization in the body. The glycocalyx is also protect the cells against dehydration and its viscosity may inhibit the nutrient movement from the cells.

- ✰ Capsulated bacteria are generally more virulent as compared to non-Capsulated bacteria.
- ✰ For demonstration of Capsule – negative staining is done with india ink.

Flagella (Flagellum - Singular)

Some bacterial species characteristically lack these motility structure, while others may possess as many as one hundred flagella (example: Proteus species). Flagella is a extremely thin hair like appendages that protrude through cell wall and originated from a basal body located beneath the cytoplasmic membrane are called flagella.

Structure of Flagella

Bacteria having flagella are motile. Each flagellum is semi-regid, helical, rotar type structure that moves the cell by rotaring from basal body.

Flagellum has three basic parts.

1. Filament
2. Hook
3. Basal body

1. Filament

It is long outer most region which is constant in diameter and contain the globular protein called flagellin, that is arranged in several chains that intertwine and form a helix around a hallow coat. Flagellin proteins are the motile protein.

2. Hook

Filament is attached to slightly vital hook consisting of a different proteins.

3. Basal Body

It is structure which anchor the flagellum to the cell wall and plasma-membrane. The basal body is composed of small central rod into a series of ring. The gram negative bacteria contain rings, the outer pair of ring is anchored to various portion of cell wall and inner pair of rings is anchored to plasma-membrane, while in gram positive bacteria only inner pair of ring is present.

The rotation of flagellum may be clockwise or anticlockwise around its axis,which results from the rotation of its basal body. This rotation pushes the bacterial cells against the surrounding liquid and propel the bacterial cell.

Flagellar protein can elicit a good antidody response in host and in these cases the flagellr protein is referred to as 'H' antigen. Somatic, cell body antigens are referred to as 'O' antigens.

Advantage of Flagella

It makes or enables the bacterium to moves towards the favorable environment or said that away from the adverse conditions.

Flagellar and somatic antigens are used for identification and classification of pathogenic bacteria. Flagella are difficult to demonstrate under ordinary light microscope. However, by special staining procedures. They can be made visible under light microscope. They can be demonstrated by dark field illumination and electron microscope.

The number and arrangement of flagella in different bacteria may varies and based on flagellar arrangement, flagellated bacteria can be divide into four gropus:

1) **Atrichous Flagella** – Bacteria having no flagella.

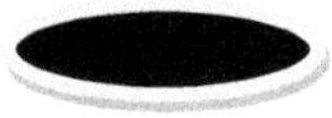

2) **Monotrichous Flagella** - Single flagellum. Example *Cholera vibrious.*

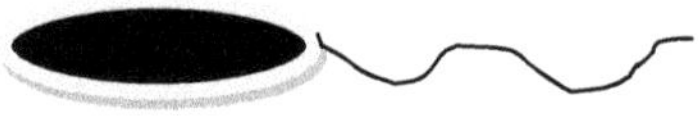

3) **Amphitrichous Flagella** – Bacteria having one flagellum at both pole example *spirillum*.

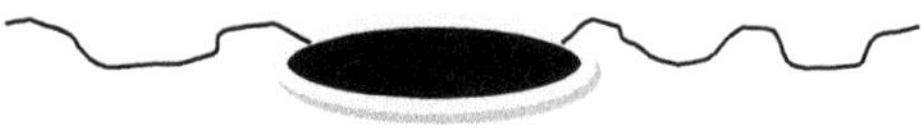

4) **Lophotrichous Flagella** – Tuft of flagella at one pole example *spirilla*.

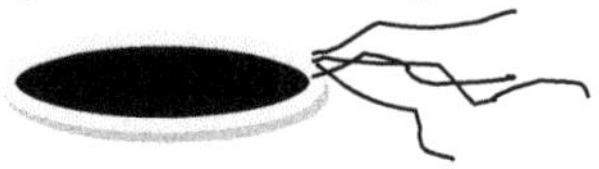

5) **Peritrichous Flagella** – Flagella may be arranged all around the cell example-typhoid bacilli, *Proteous.*

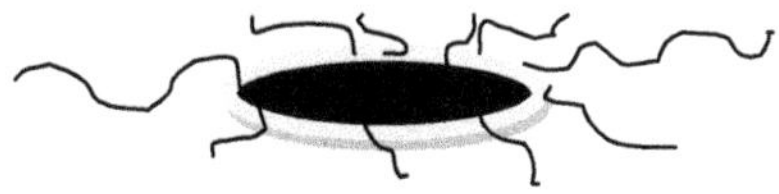

Axial Filament

The spirochates moves by the axial filaments or endo-flagella. They are bundles of fibers that arises at the ends of cell beneath the outer sheath and spirall around the cell. The axial filaments are anchor at one ends and have a structure similar to the flagella. The rotation of filament produces a movement of outer sheath and moves the spirochetes in spiral motion. Example- *Borrelia, Treponema pallidum etc.*

Fimbriae and Pili

These are straighter, thinner and shorter than flagella (about 0.5μm long and less than 10nm thick). They are made up of repeating subunit proteins via a monomer aggregation mechanism. Both the structure is anchored in the cytoplasmic membrane. Fimbriae are important structure of bacterial pathogenesis. This basic function is their attachment of bacterial cells. The number of pili per bacterium may varies from 100 to 400. The pili consist of a protein called **pilin**, which is arranged helically around the central coat. The fimbriae can occur at the pole of bacterial cell or they may be evenly distributed over the entire surface of the cell. The fimbriae help to attachment and colonization of bacteria on host surface. The pili are usually larger than fimbriae and their number is only 1 or 2 per cent, they are sometimes also called the sexpili because they join the bacterial cells in preparation for the transfer of genetic material from one cell to another.

Spore

Under un-favourable condition like starvation some bacterial cells transform themselves into spores like Bacillus and Clostridium have the ability to form resistant resting stages called spores. These are dormant forms of the organism that are resistant to high temperatures, radiation, drying and chemicals because of very low water content and high concentration of dipicolinic acid in complex association with calcium.

Under favourable condition, the calcium dipicolinate diffuses out and the spores germinate restoring heat sensitivity. Exosporum is the outermost layer of spore and consist of lipoproteins and carbohydrates. Exosporum surrounds the spore coat, which consists of insoluble structural protein and protect the spores from toxogenic substances. Inside the spore coat is a thick cortex of peptidoglycon and inner most is the cell wall, consisting of normal cell wall components.

Spore of all medically important species are destroyed by autoclaving temperature at 120°C – 15lb – 15 minutes.

The transformation of a bacterial cell to the spore state is a differentiation process through several distinct stages.

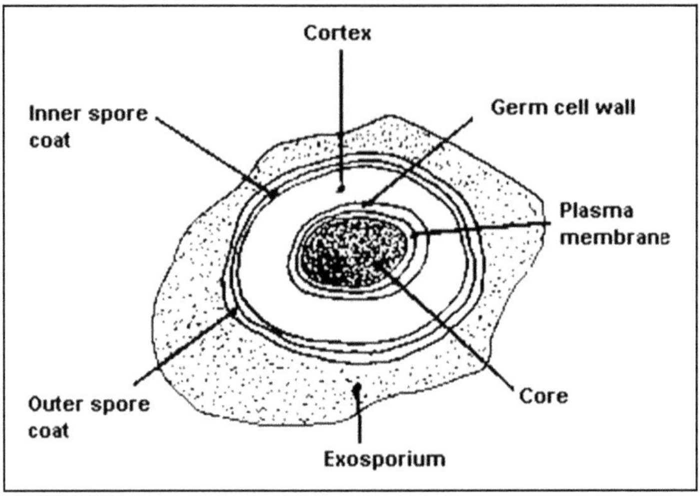

Figure 4.5: Structure of Bacterial Endo-spore.

Spores having different size and shapes depending on their location in the bacterial cell.

Different size and shape

- Central — Exp. *Bacillus anthracis*
- Sub terminal — *Clostridium chauvoei*
- Terminal
  - Spherical — *Cl.tetani*
  - Ovoid — *Cl.tertium*

Chapter 5

Bacterial Nutrition and Growth

Introduction

Microorganisms require nutrients to obtain energy and to construct new cellular components as well as its multiplication. Some mineral elements are required in traces. Some factors like as temperature, oxygen level and osmotic concentration of the medium play critical role in cultivation of bacteria aids in the control of microbial growth and the study of ecological distribution of microorganisms.

Nutrients Requirements

Bacteria require a balanced mixture of nutrients and divided into two major groups.

1. **Macronutrients -** Macronutrients are required in relatively large amounts, *e.g.* Carbon, oxygen, hydrogen, nitrogen, sulphure, phosphorus, calcium and magnesium. The first six components (C, O, H, N, S and P) are components of carbohydrates, lipids, proteins and nucleic acids. The remaining compounds exist in the cell as cations. Carbon is needed for the backbone or skeleton of all organic molecules.
2. **Micronutrients -** Micronutrients are required in small amounts, *e.g.* manganese, zinc, cobalt, molybdenum, nickel, copper and iron. These are the part of enzymes and co-factors, and help in catalysis of reactions and maintenance of protein structure.

Growth Factors

Growth factors are required by bacteria because they are essential cell components. There are four major classes of Growth factors - Amino acid (For protein synthesis), purine and pyrimidine (For nucleic acids synthesis),vitamins (For enzymes cofactors), and heme (For hemoglobin and cytochrome).

The principal constituent of bacterial cells is water, which represents around 80 per cent of the total weight. Water is also required for hydrolytic reactions carried out by the cell.

Bacteria can be classified nutritionally, based on their energy requirements and on their ability to synthesize essential metabolites.

- ☆ **Phototrophs** – Bacteria which derived their energy from sunlight
- ☆ **Chemotrophs** – Bacteria can obtain energy from chemical reactions.
- ☆ **Autotrophs** – Bacteria that can synthesize all their organic compounds called autotrophs.
- ☆ **Heterotrophs** – Bacteria that are unable to synthesize their own metabolites and depends on preformed organic compounds are called heterotrophs.

Autotrophs are able to utilize atmospheric carbon dioxide and nitrogen. Whereas heterotrophic bacteria are unable to grow with carbon dioxide as the sole source of carbon.

Growth and Multiplication of Bacteria

Bacteria are divided by binary fission process. In this process the bacterial cell grows almost double in its original size. A transverse septum across the cell and divide the parent cell into two daughter cells. This rate of cell division differ among bacteria. It is depend on the species of bacteria, age of the culture medium, nutrient content of the medium, temperature, carbon dioxide concentration and many other factors. In some species, the daughter cells may remain partially attach after division.

Generation Time (Population Doubling Time)

It is the time required for a cells to divided (its population to double) called **Generation Time.** It varies considerably among organisms and with environmental condition like as temperature *etc.* Most bacteria have Generation Time f 1-3 hrs but it may be as little as 20 minutes (*e.g. E.coli*) and may be 15-20 hours (*e.g. Mycobacterium tuberculosis*). If a binary fission is continue unchecked and enormous number of cells will be produced, if a doubling occurred every 20 minutes after 20 generation, a single cell could increase to over million cells, and this is required as little as 7 hours of times. In 30th generation/10 hours, the population would be one billion and similarly in 24 hours, the number could be 10^{21} because of this type of growth pattern, the growth of bacteria being exponential, is expressed in the log values. When a bacterial population is continue to grow in a slant or liquid medium, there is limited nutrient which is absorbed by bacteria and further their accumulation of toxic product of metabolism as a consequence the rate of growth declines and eventually growth stops.

Generation Time Formula

Generation Time (t) = t log2/log B_t – log B_o

where,

t = Time interval in minutes

B_o = No. of cells at beginning time

B_t = No. of cells after time interval

Generation time varies with species and depends on

1. Concentration of available nutrients in medium
2. Temperature of the incubation
3. Supply of oxygen for aerobes
4. pH
5. Metabolites produced by bacteria, sometimes

Bacterial Growth Curve

Growth is defined as increase in cellular constituents and may result in an increase in a microorganism's size, population numbers or both.

The growth curve of bacteria can be divided into four phases.

1. Lag Phase or Adjacent Phase
2. Log Phase or exponential growth Phase
3. Stationary Phase or Equillibrium Phase
4. Decline or Death Phase

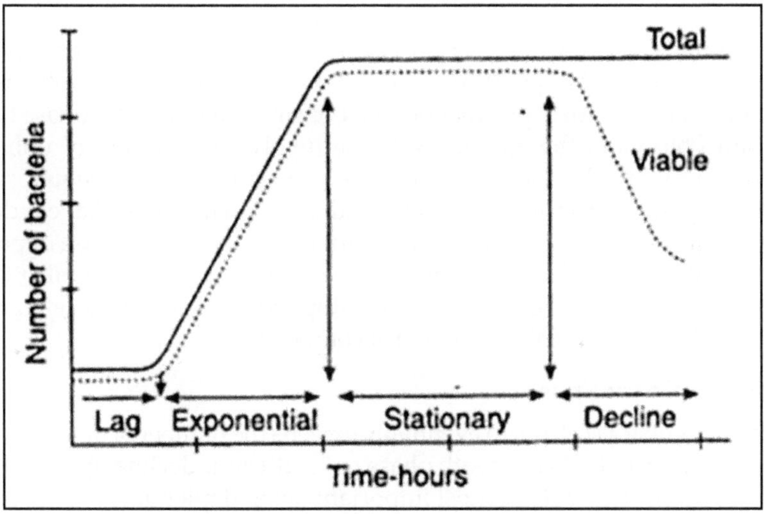

Figure 5.1: Bacterial Growth Curve.

1. Lag Phase or Adjacent Phase

When the bacterial cells are inoculated in a fresh culture medium usually no immediate increase in cell number occurs. This period of adjacent is called as Lag Phase or when the cells are transferred from a culture of a stationary phase to a fresh medium, the bacterial cells undergo a change of chemical composition therefore they are capable of initiating the growth. This period no cell division is called Lag Phase. Lag Phase is extremely variable in duration depends upon the conditions of the microorganisms. It can be few hours or several days. However the cells are not dormant during this time they undergo a period of intense metabolic activity.

2. Log Phase or Exponential Growth Phase/Multiplication Phase

After the phase of adjustment the cells begins to divide and enter into a period of growth or logrithimic increase, which is called as Log Phase or exponential growth Phase. In this phase, there is exponential relationship between the number of cells in the population and time. The cellular reproduction is most active during this period and population number doubles at a constant rate called **generation time**. In this phase, cells are more active metabolically and the products of the cells are most efficient and that's why log phase cells are preferred for industrial purpose. However during log phase of growth microorganism are highly sensitive to adverse condition like radiation and antimicrobial drugs. This phase is used for biochemical and physiological studies.

3. Stationary Phase or Equillibrium Phase

If the exponential growth continued unchecked, there will be a large population of bacterial cells could arises which practically not take places. The growth rate eventually slows down. Number of microbial death balances the number of new cells and population stabilizes. The metabolic activity of individuals survival cells also slow at this stage. This is a period of equillibrium as called Stationary Phase. The growth of bacterial population is limited by exhaustion of available nutrient or by accumulation of toxic product of metabolism. The transition phase between equilibrium Phase and the Stationary Phase involve in a period of unbalanced growth during which various cellular factor are synthesize at unequal rate and due to this imbalanced growth, the cells in the stationary phase have a different chemical composition. The cellular composition of cells in this phase depends on specific growth, limiting factors despite this, cells of this phase are smaller than the exponential phase because cell division has stopped and secondary cells are more resistant to adverse physical and chemical composition.

4. Decline or Death Phase

There is number of cell death eventually exceeds the number of new cells formed and the population enter in the death phase or logathrimic decline phase. The death results from number of factors, most important being depletion of cellular reserve of the energy. Similar to growth death is also a exponential function and hence in a logathrimic plot the death phase is lenear decrease in the number of viable cells with time. The death rate is also highly variable because its depends on environment and characteristic of the organism.

Measurement of Bacterial Growth

There are varieties of techniques used for the measurement of bacterial growth. (Total count and viable count).

a) Measurement of Cell Numbers

The cell number can be determining by.

I) Direct counting methods- By using Petroff-hausser counting chamber, Electronic cell counter and by hemocytometers.

II) Direct counting methods- By colony count includes Pour plate method, spread plate method and by dilution techniques, simple sensitive and most widely used for viable counts.

b) Measurement of Cell Mass

Increase in cell mass and cell number accompanies population growth. So measurement of cell mass can be used to detect growth. Techniques are:

I) By Measurement of wet and dry weight of bacteria.

II) By determination of the turbidity of the culture using Brown's opacity tube and a photoelectric colorimeter or spectrophotometer.

III) By measuring total nitrogen contents.

The Influence of Environmental Factors on Growth

The growth of bacteria is affected by the physical and chemical nature of the surrounding.

H-ion Concentration

The bacteria are sensitive to variation in the Ph. Each species of bacteria has a pH range, in above or below pH bacteria does not survive. The majority of most pathogenic bacteria grow best on pH 7.2-7.6. Acidophiles have their optimum growth between pH range of 0 and 5.5, Neutrophiles between 5.508.0 and alkalophiles between pH ranges of 8.5-11.5. Drastic variation in cytoplasmic pH can harm bacteria by disrupting the plasma-membrane or inhibiting the enzymes activity and membrane transport proteins.

Temperature

It is one of the most important factors for growth of bacteria. On the basis of temperature requirements bacteria can be sub-divided into four groups...

I) Psychrophilic (Gk Psychros - Cold, philein - Love) = Temperature range from 0 – 20°C

Habitate - Tissue of cold blooded animals.

II) Mesophilic (Gk Meso – intermediate, philein – Love) =

Temperature range from 20 – 45°C

Habitate - Tissue of man, animals and birds.

III) Thermophilic (Gk Thermos – Warm, philein – Love) =

Temperature range from 45 – 55°C

Habitate - Top layers of soil, hot spring and manure.

IV) Hyperthermophilic -Temperature range from 85 – 100°C

c) Light and Radiations

Except phototropic bacteria are grow well in dark, high energy or short wave-length radiations harms in many ways. X- rays and gamma rays- ions molecules and destroy DNA and other cell components. U.V-radiation can break DNA strands exposure to light may influence pigment production.

d) Osmotic Effect

Most bacteria are hypertonic to the habitat. The amount of water actually available to bacteria is expressed water activity. Although most bacteria will not grow well at water activity 0.98 due to plasmolysis and associated effects. Osmotolerant bacteria survive and grow well. Halophiles require high concentration of sodium chloride.

e) Oxygen Requirement

Based on gaseous requirement bacteria can be categorized as obligate aerobes, obligate anaerobes, facultative anaerobes and microaerophiles.

Chapter 6

Sterilization and Disinfection

Introduction

Sterilization is the free of an article from all living organisms including viable spores. In this process kills more than 10^6 organisms, including spores of a defined, exceptionally high degree of resistance.

Disinfection is the freeing of an article from vegetative form of pathogenic microorganisms, but not their endospores. Disinfection is the only convenient procedure for floors, bench tops, washbasins and other large surface in the laboratory.

Method of Sterilization

The methods include heat, chemical, filtration and radiation.

1. Heat

Heat is the most generally applicable and reliable method of sterilization. It should be used wherever possible. The bacterial cell protoplasm is composed of proteins distributed well balance in colloidal state. When applied heat, there protein coagulate, which result in the death of the cell.

Various factors that can be considered for sterilization by heat are:

a) Thermal Death Point (TDP)

Lowest temperature at which all the organisms in liquid suspension will be killed in 10 minutes.

b) *Thermal Death Time (TDT)*

The minimum length of time in which all the bacteria will be killed at a given temperature. TDP and TDT are guideline that indicate the severity of treatment required to kill a population of bacteria.

c) *Decimal Reduction Time (DRT)*

Time in minutes, in which 90 per cent of the population of bacteria will be killed.

1.1 Dry Heat

This method kills the bacteria due to protein denaturation, oxidative damage and toxic effects of elevated levels of electrolyte.

Following are the various methods of dry heat sterilization.

I) Red Heat

This has its main application in the sterilization of inoculating wire and loops. These should be heald almost vertically in a Bunsen flame, until red hot, along its whole length. Point of forceps, needles, scissors etc may also be heated until red.

II) Direct Flaming

In this, process articles are passed over flame 3-4 times without allowing it to become red hot. Direct flaming is done for the sterilization of mouth of culture tubes, cotton plugs and glass slide *etc.*

III) Hot Air Sterilization

Heating by exposure to hot air is an accepted method for the sterilization of articles that cannot be reliably penetrated by steam and can tolerate the high temperatures required *e.g.* 160°C -180°C. Here sterilization is done by application of dry heat. It kills the organisms by oxidizing their chemical constituents. Hot air is less effective than moist heat and less penetrating.

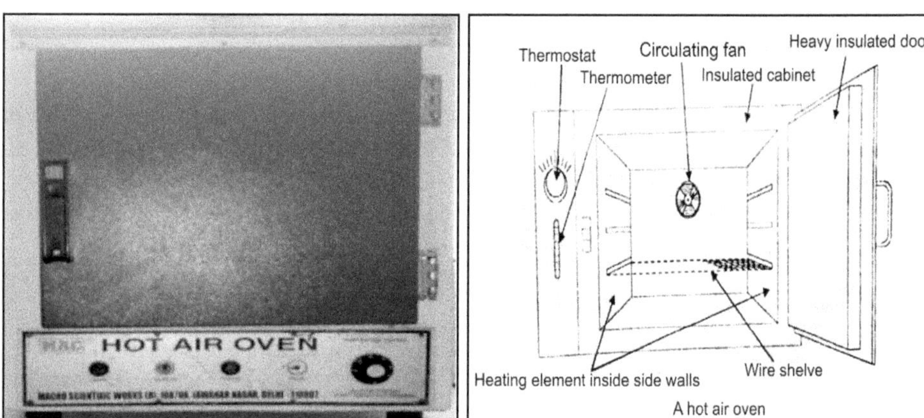

Figure 6.1: Hot Air Oven.

Hot air oven is used for sterilization of glassware as tubes, flasks, measuring cylinder, all glass syringes and glass pipettes. Metal instruments may also be sterilized by hot air.

It is a cuboidal or rectangular metallic chamber fitted with heating elements, a thermostat for temperature regulation and a fan for uniform distribution of heat throughout the chamber. The inner space of the chamber is fitted with racks.

1.2. Moist Heat

Most heat kills the bacteria by denaturation and coagulation of proteins. The most commonly used method for moist heat is autoclave. In this sterilized all kind of bacteriological media, rubber goods, laboratory coats and aprons *etc.* The autovlave temperature is 121°C – 15lb pressure for 15 minutes in this temperature all the vegetative bacterial cells and spores are destroyed.

Table 6.1: Method of Sterilization

Method	*Use*	*Limitations*
	Physical Agents for Sterilization	
☆ **Dry heat**		
Hot air oven	Sterilizing materials impermeable to or damage by moisture	Material which cannot sustained the high temperature for long time
Incineration	Disposal of contaminated objects that cannot be again uses	Size of inceratior must be adequate to burn large loads promptly and completely, potential of air pollution.
☆ **Moist heat**		
Autoclave	Sterilizing surgical instruments, surgical trays, utensils, media and other liquid material.	Ineffective against organisms in material impervious to steam, cannot be used for heat sensitive articles.
By steam or boiling water	Destruction of non-spore forming pathogenic organisms.	No guaranteed to produce sterilization on one exposure.
☆ **Radiation**		
Ultra-violet light	To control air born infection and disinfection of working area.	Must be absorbed to be effective (not pass the glass), irritation in eyes and skin.
Radiation by X-rays and gamma rays	Sterilization of surgical material which are sensitive to heat	Expensive and technical requirements.
☆ **Filtration**		
By membrane filters	Sterilization of heat sensitive biological material	Fluid must be relatively free of suspended particular matter.
☆ **Physical method**		
Washing	Objects, hand and skin	Sanitizes, reduces microbial flora

2. Moist Heat

2.1 Below 100°C

I) Pasteurization

It is the process of killing bacteria at below boiling point temperature. This method is used for sterilization of milk. On the basis of time and temperature requirement, two method used for the pasteurization.

Holding Method

In this method, pasteurization is done in 145°F temperature for the 30 minutes.

Flash Method

In this method, pasteurization is done in 160°F temperature for the 15 seconds.

Above both the methods are sufficient to kill the vegetative bacterial cells but not sufficient for bacterial spores.

2.2 Boiling at 100°C

I) Tyndallization

It is the process of sterilization of bacteriological media by keeping the medium at 100°C in flowing steam for 30 minutes and for three successive days with intermittent incubation. This method is also known as 'fractional sterilization'spore that survive the initial heating heating may be expected to germinate in the medium, during intermittent incubation and the resulting vegetative bacteria will be killed when the medium is reheated.

II) Serum Inspissator

Inspissation is a procedure of fractional by moist heat at lower temperature. In the method the media is exposed to a temperature of 80°C for three successive days with intermittent incubation. An inspisstor is a water-jacketed copper box. A thermostate regulates the temperature. The inspissator is mainly used for sterilization heat labile

Egg medium, serum media and sugar media.

2.3 Steaming Above 100°C

I) Autoclave

The most effective and reliable method of sterilization is by steam under pressure. It is usually sufficient to expose the material for 15 minutes at 15 lb pressure (psi). This will accomplish a temperature of 121°C that kill all the bacteria and their spores, viruses, fungi and protozoa. Steam sterilization is more effective than dry heat because steam easily and rapidly penetrate to all parts of the vessel.

Autoclaving is a reliable method of sterilizing culture media and other laboratory supplies. It should be used for all materials that are water containing, permeable or wettable and not liable to be damaged by the process. Most of the culture media, aprons, bandages, surgical instruments, syringes, rubber appliances, discards etc are safely and effectively sterilized by steam under pressure. Sugar, fats and oils cannot be sterilized in autoclave at usual temperature and pressure.

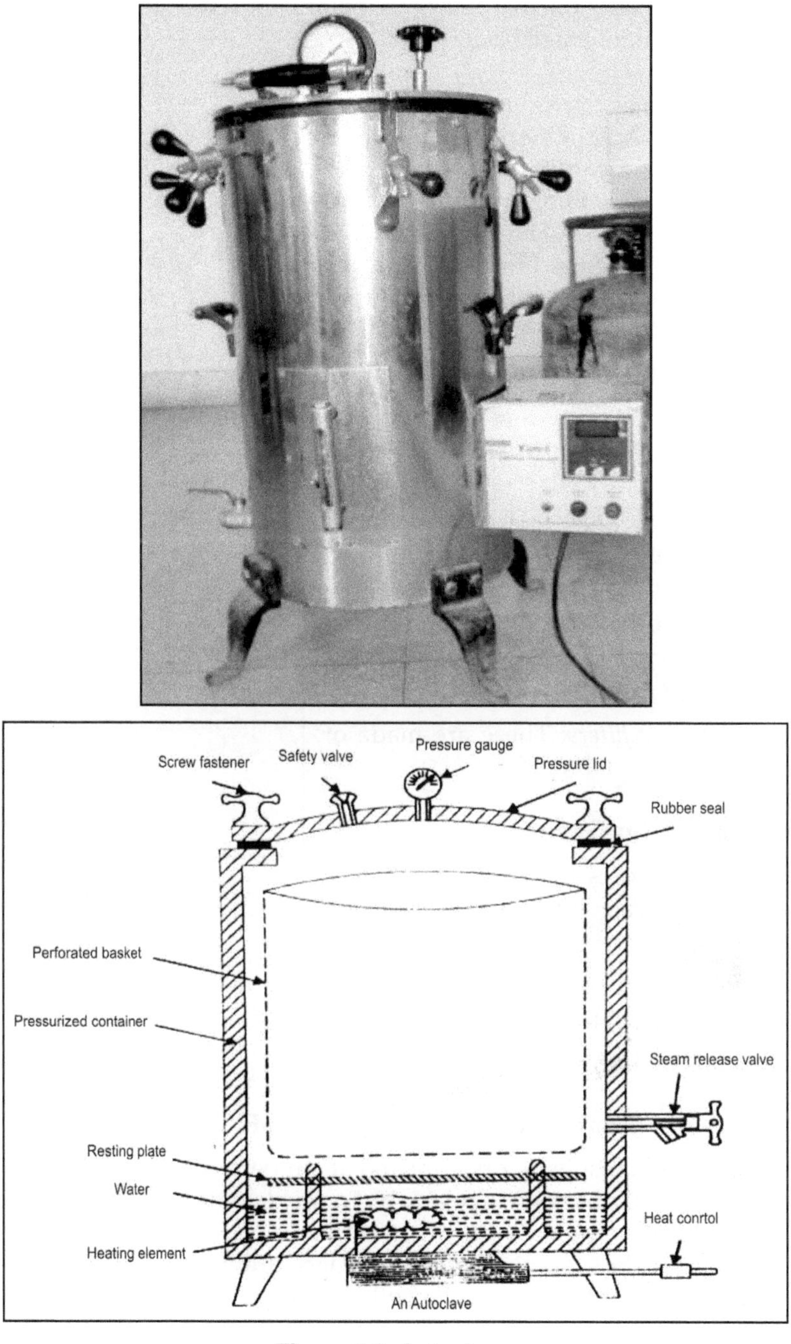

Figure 6.2: Autoclave.

II) Boiling

Commonly used for sterilization of needles and syringes *etc.* Most of the vegetative bacterial cells are killed at 50 to 70°C with in short period of time. Many bacterial spores are also killed at 100°C. So, boiling for few minutes is sufficient to make free from contaminated bacteria.

3. Filtration

This is the method of sterilization of heat labile liquids such as antibiotics, serum and organic substance containing medium *etc.* It is also used to remove bacterial cells from toxin. There are various types of filters is available, filter is of different pore size and thir used depening upon the viscosity of the liquids.

The commonly used **microbiological filters** are:

a) Seitz filters: These are made of asbestos pads.

b) Sintered glass filters: These are made of fused porus glass.

c) Chamberland and Selas candle type filters: These are made of unglazed porcelain.

d) Berkefeld and Mandler filters: These are made of diatomaceous earth.

e) Membrane filters: These are made of cellulose membrane.

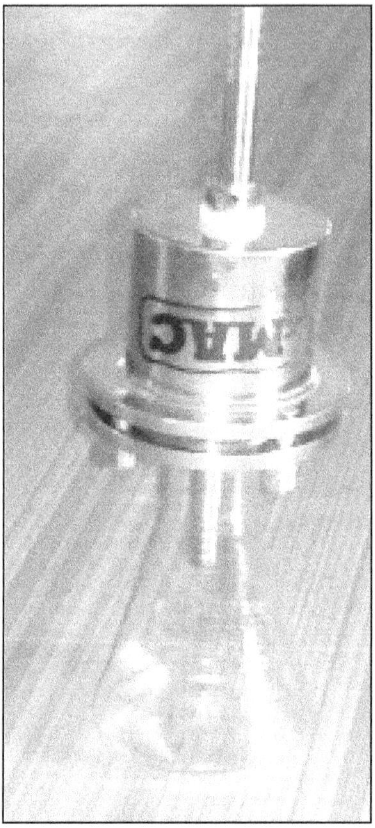

Figure 6.3: Procedure of Filtration.

4. Sterilization by Gases

A number of processes are used for the gas sterilization of delicate, heat labile equipment. These are:

a) Exposure to low-temperature steam and formaldehyde (LTSF)

b) Exposure to ethylene oxide

c) Exposure to gas plasma

Low-Temperature Steam and Formaldehyde (LTSF)

Steam at sub-atmospheric pressure and at temperature below 100°C kills the spores of thermophillic bacteria very slowly. Formaldehyde is sporicidal substance, but only at high concentration in the presence of moisture. Together, formaldehyde and steam appear to be synergistic. Very low concentration of formaldehyde gas in the presence of sub-atmospheric steam will kill spores. Formaldehyde is toxic and irritates eyes and respiratory tract at concentrations above 2ppm.

5. Sterilization by Radiation

Radiation has various effects on the cell depending upon its wavelength, intensity and duration.

Types

a) Ionizing radiation

b) Non- Ionizing radiation

a) Ionizing Radiation

Ionizing radiations are such as gamma rays, X- rays or high energy electron beam, has a wavelength shorter than non-ionizing radiations *i.e.* >1 nm. Therefore it carries more energy.

Gamma rays are emitted by radioactive cobalt and electron beam is produced by accelerating electron to high energies in special machine.

Gamma radiations penetrate deeply but requires long time for sterilization of large masses. High energy electron beam have much less penetration power but require less time of exposure.

Principle effect of this radiation is ionization of water molecules, which forms highly reactive hydroxyl radicals. These hydroxyl radicals react with cellular organic components of DNA and kill them.

This is used for sterilization of plastic wares, dental and medical supplies.

b) Non-Ionizing radiations

Non- ionizing radiation has a longer wavelength than ionizing radiation, usually < 1nm. For examples ultra violet light damage the DNA of exposed cells by causing the bonds to be formed between adjacent thymine in DNA chain. These thymine dimmers inhibit correct replication of DNA during reproduction of cell. Ultraviolet at a wavelength of 260 nm is more effective for killing organism because it is absorbed maximum by the cellular DNA. Ultraviolet lamps or germicidal lamps are used in the laboratory and hospitals.

Disinfection

Disinfection is a process, which is effective principally on non-acid fast vegetative organism. Its action on bacterial endospores is uncertain.

OR

Disinfection defined as the "destruction of microorganisms but not bacterial spores" reduces the microbial population at safe level.

OR

Disinfections are chemical agents that may kill vegetative bacteria, fungi, and viruses and occasionally, spore by the destruction of proteins, lipid and nucleic acids in the cell or its cytoplasmic membrane.

Factors Affecting the Activity of Disinfectant

a) The concentration of chemical agents used.
   Lower concentration – act as bacteriostatic not act as bacteriocidal.
b) The temperature at which the agent is being used. Generally the lower the temperature, the lower the effectiveness.
c) pH of the media.
d) Duration of application
e) The number of the microorganisms present. The more microorganisms present the harder to eliminate.
f) Duration of application
g) The nature of the material bearing the microorganisms. Organic material such as dirt and excreta interfere with some agents.

Type of Disinfectant

1) Phenol and phenolics
2) Chlorohexidine
3) Halogens
4) Iodophore
5) Chlorine
6) Alcohals
7) Heavy metals and their compounds
8) Surface acting agents
a) Soaps
9) Quaternary Ammonium compounds
10) Organic acid derivatives
11) Aldehydes
12) Gaseous chemosterilizers
13) Oxidizing agent

1) Phenol and Phenolics

Phenol (carbolic acid) used earlier, is not be used now days because of its odour and irritation to skin. Phenolics are the derivative of phenol. Phenolics are a chemically altered compounds so that to reduce irritation and also increase the antimicrobial activity to injured plasma membrane, inactivate the enzymes and denature the proteins. Most commonly used phenolics is cresol (*O*-Phenyl phenol) used in the formation of Lysol.

2) Chlorohexidine

It is used for disinfecting the skin and mucous membrane and skin in combination with detergents or alcohol. It is kills the bacteria by damage the plasma-membrane and also effective against viruses.

3) Halogens

Halogens compounds like chlorine and iodine in alone or with the combination of other compounds are act strong antimicrobial agents.

- ☆ Iodine is a most effective antiseptic; its action is that it combines with tyrosine amino-acid, enzymes and cellular protein. Iodine also oxidized the –SH group of amino-acids that are required for to maintain protein structure.

4) Iodophore

It is combination of iodine plus inorganic molecules in which iodine is released slowly *e.g.* Betadine, isodine and tincture iodine used for skin disinfectant and wound treatment.

5) Chlorine

Chlorine is a gas and with the other compound combination used as used as disinfectant. Its germicidal action is caused by hypochlorus acid (HOCl) that is formed when chlorine is added to water.It inhibit the cellular enzyme system function *e.g.* Disinfect the drinking water, sewage *etc.*

6) Alcohals

Alcohal is control the microbial activity by killing the bacteria and fungi but not to endospores and viruses (non-enveloped). It is usually denaturing the protein but in the enveloped viruses it dissolve the lipid components and disrupt the membrane. Ethanol and isopropenol is most commonly used alcohols.

7) Heavy Metals and their Compounds

Heavy metals like silver, mercury and copper act as an antiseptic or germicidal. When metals ions combines with –SH groups on cellular protein, resulting denaturation occur.

Mercuric chloride – it is antiseptic and its use is limited because of its toxicity, corressiveness and in effectiveness in organic matter.

Copper in the form of copper sulphate is used to destroy algae.

8) Surface Acting Agents

a) Soaps

Soap has little value of antiseptic agents. There is mechanically remove the microorganisms by scrubbing.

Sanitizers are important in cleaning of utensils and dairy equipments. They are non-toxic, non-corrosive and fast acting.

9) Quaternary Ammonium Compounds

Quaternary Ammonium compounds (Quats) are bactericidal against gram positive and gram negative bacteria. This compound effect on the bacterial plasma membrane permeability and resulting loss of cytoplsmic constituents.

10) Organic Acid Derivatives

Thre is number of organic acid derivatives such as sorbic acid and benzoic acid used for the food disinfection.

11) Aldehydes

Most commonly used aldehydes are formaldehyde and glutaraldehydes.

Formaldehyde - used for the specimen preservation, bacterial inactivation and in vaccines.

Glutaraldehydes – bactericidal action and used in equipment sterilization and hospital disinfectant.

12) Gaseous Chemosterilizers

Gaseous chemosterilizers is used to sterilize the close chamber for aseptical work and most commonly used gas is ethylene oxide and less commonly used gases are propylene oxide and β - propiolactone. This gas cause denaturation of the bacterial protein which ultimately kill the microbes. *e.g.* Sterilization of disposable plasticwares.

13) Oxidizing Agent

Oxidizing agent has antimicrobial activity by affecting the cellular component of the microorganisms. The most commonly used oxidisizing agents are hydrogen paraoxide (H_2O_2)and ozone. hydrogen paraoxide (H_2O_2) is effective for sterilization of inanimate objects whereas ozone with chlorine used for water disinfectant.

Table 6.2: Common Antiseptics and Disinfectants

Antiseptics	*Disinfectants*	
☆ Chlorhexadine acetate	☆ Alkyl dimethyl-chloride benzyl ammonium	☆ Glutaraldehyde
☆ Chlorhexadine digluconate	☆ Ammonium chloride	☆ O-benzyl-p-chlorophenol
☆ Iodine complex	☆ Chlrohexidine diacetate	Octyl decyl dimethyl ammonium chloride
☆ Isopropyl alcohol	☆ Chlrohexidine gluconate	☆ Orthophenyl phenol
☆ Isopropranol	☆ Chlorine	☆ Phosphoric acid
☆ Polyalkyleneglycol-iodine/ Potassium iodide	Dioctyl dimethyl ammonium chloride	P-tert-amylphenol
☆ Povidine- iodine	☆ Iodine	☆ Quaternary ammonium
☆ Titrable-iodine	Dioctyl dimethyl ammonium chloride	☆ Sodium o- benzyle-p-chloro-phenate
	☆ Ethyl alcohol	☆ O-phenyl-phenate
	☆ Formaldehyde	☆ P-tertiary amyl phenate
		☆ Synthetic phenol

Table 6.3: Disinfectant and their Mode of Application

Target	*Disinfectant*	*Strength to Use (Disinfectant/ Material V/V)*	*Application*	*Time of Exposure*
Skin	Ethanol	70 per cent	Direct	2 Minutes
	Iodine	1 per cent	Direct	2 Minutes
	Povidine iodine	per cent 1	Direct	2 Minutes
	Quats		Direct	2 Minutes
Blood	Cresol	5 per cent	2:01	6 hours
	Ca hypochlorite	1 per cent	2:01	6 hours
Urine	Cresol (pH 9.0)	5 per cent	1:01	4 hours
Sputum	Cresol (pH 9.0)	5 per cent	1:01	4 hours
Faeces	Cresol(pH9)	5 per cent	2:01	6 hours
	Hypochlorite	1 per cent	3:01	6 hours
	Ca hydroxide	20 per cent	2:01	6 hours
Glassware	Hypochlorite	1 per cent	Direct	4 hours
Laboratory instruments	Hypochlorite	0.1 per cent	Direct	4 hours
	Isopropanol	70 per cent	Direct	4 hours
Work benches	Lysol	5 per cent	Direct	4 hours
	Cresol	1 per cent	Direct	4 hours
	Hypochlorite	5 per cent	Direct	4 hours
	Chloramine		Direct	4 hours

Chapter 7

Disease, Source and Transmission of Infection

Introduction

The animals are susceptible for many infections caused by microorganisms. Some microorganisms can invade animal tissues and resist defenses by producing various enzymes or products likes' toxins that can seriously affect the health. Balance exists between defenses and disease producing organisms and animals remain healthy but when this balance is disturbed microorganisms overpower the defenses system and disease is occurring.

Definition

Pathogens – Pathogens are organism, which can invade the body, multiply and produce disease. The disease is occur, when balance between defense and disease producing organisms is disturbed (or overcome the defense capabilities). Disease is occurring.

Infection - A disease state due to the invasion or colonization of body by pathogenic bacteria.

Disease - It occur when infection bring any change from the state of health. It means disease is an abnormal state in which a body part or all of the body is not able to function properly.

Host – An organism that shelters and supports the growth of microorganisms.

Microbiota/Normal microflora –The microorganisms that lives in the body but do not produce any disease under normal condition are called Normal microflora.

Relationship between Normal Microflora and Host Microbial Antagonism

Normal flora can prevent the over growth of harmful microorganisms as there are completion for the nutrients. Microflora also produces conditions which are harmful to the invading microbes by lower pH and oxygen availability, production of antimicrobial substances like bactericin (*E. coli* in intestine) that inhibit the growth of *Salmonella* and *Shigella*.

Forms of Symbiosis (Symbiosis = Living together)

State in which there is specialized and beneficial relationship between host and microorganisms.

Symbiosis has different forms:

a) Commensalism – One of the host is benefited and other is not affected. They remain in or on the body surface without harming the host.
b) Mutualism – In this, organism and the host receive mutual benefit.
c) Parasitism- In this, organism lives at the expense of the host and cause harm to the host.

Classification of Infection according to the Source

1. **Primary infection-**Initial infection of host with the organism.
2. **Secondary infection-**Primary infection along with the invasion of another species of organisms.
3. **Reinfection-**Subsequent infection by same organisms.
4. **Cross infection-**Individual suffering from one infectious disease and get a infection from another host.
5. **Nosocomial infection-**Infection that acquired in hospital.
6. **Subclinical or asymptomatic infection-** There is clinical sign are absent but causative agent continue to multiply.
7. **Acute infection-**Infection is characterized by sudden onset and short course.
8. **Chronic infection-** Slowly progressive infection with the shedding of etiological agents.
9. **Latent infection-** In this, during infection causative agent is not possible to isolates.

Classification of Infectious Disease

Symptoms – Change in the body function like pain and discomfort. These changes are not apparently observed by observer.

Signs – Changes, which are apparent and a patient can exhibit. These changes can observe by observer.

Syndrome – Specific group of symptoms or signs accompanying a particular disease.

Communicable disease – Any disease that spreads from one host to another directly or indirectly. *e.g.* FMD, Pox in animal

Contagious disease – Disease spread very easily from one person to another *e.g.* Chicken pox in man.

Non- Communicable disease – Disease that does not spreads from one host to another. *e.g.* Tetanus by *Clostridium tetani*

Incidence of disease – It is the fraction of population that contracts the disease during a particular period. Occurrence of a disease in a population.

Prevalence of disease – It is the fraction of population that contract the disease during specified time.

Sporadic disease – When disease occurs occasionally like tetanus.

Endemic disease – When disease is present constantly in a population like common cold.

Epidemic disease – Many people in a given area acquire certain disease in a relatively short period.

Pandemic disease – An epidemic disease, which occurs world wide *e.g. Influenza.*

Acute disease – A disease, which develops rapidly butlosts only for short period *e.g. Influenza.*

Chronic disease – It develop slowly, body reaction is less severe but disease is likely to continue for long period *e.g. Tuberculosis.*

Latent disease – It is disease in which the disease producing organism remains inactive for a time then become active and produce a disease after sometime.

Local infection – When an invading microorganisms are limited to a small area of body *e.g.* Abscess.

Systemic infection – When microorganisms are spread throughout the body.

Bacterimia – Bacteria are present in blood known as bacterimia

Septicemia – When bacteria multiply in the blood.

Toxemia – Presence of toxin in the blood.

Viremia – Virus present in the blood.

Source of Infection and Method of Transmission of Infectious Agents

The major sources of organisms, which are involved in disease producing, are animals and less common source are inanimate objects.

a) **Animals self as a sources of microorganism** – In a animals, normal flora are present, which consist of microorganisms. These microorganisms are opportunistic and capable to produce disease under certain circumstances. The microbial flora commonly present in different parts of the body includes bacteria, yeast and fungi.

b) **Incubation stage of disease or Period of incubation** – Incubation period, it is period from the entry of the pathogenic organism to develop the clinical sign. During this period the animal is discharging disease producing organisms. In the respiratory and intestinal disease, causative agents are shed during incubation period.

c) **Animal with clinical symptoms** – Such types of animal who show clinical symptoms usually shed large number of organisms. The route of excretion of the organisms is depends upon the nature of the disease. The duration of shedding of the organisms is varies with different diseases.

   Acute disease – Shedding of organisms is for short duration.

   Chronic disease – Shedding of organisms is for long duration.

d) **Animal with sub-clinical infection** – Carrier animals does not show clinical symptoms (but having the pathogenic bacteria), carrier state of animals is also depends upon the immune status of animal and pathogenicity of the disease. Such types of animals are infected or spread the disease to others animals by secretion or excretion.

e) **Animals at convalescent carrier stage or Period of convalescent** - After clinical recovery some of the animals, shed organism for a varying period of time (convalescent stage). In anthrax in cattle, there is no convalescent stage.

Transmission of Disease

The causative agent of the disease can be transmitted from reservoir of infection to susceptible host by three main/major routes:

a) Contact Transmission

I) **Direct transmission** -Disease is transmitted from one individual to other by physical contact between its source and susceptible host *e.g.* *Staphylococcus* infection.

II) **In-Direct transmission** - When the agent of the disease is transmitted via non-living object. The non-living object is known as fomite, towel and surgical instruments.

III) **Droplet transmission** –Organisms are discharged in air by coughing, sneezing, laughing *etc.*

b) Vehicle Transmission

Causative agent is transmitted by water, food, air born *etc.*

c) Vector Transmission

Causative agent is transmitted from one host to another via. arthropod vectors.

I) **Mechanical transmission -** Causative agent is transmitted mechanically (via. Insects) *e.g.* Typhoid. It is passive transport of pathogens.

II) **Biological transmission –** It is active transport and arthropod bites the animal and might ingest some of the infected blood. The pathogen is reproduced in some arthropod and increase in number. Arthropod can transmit the organisms/pathogens via bite or deification, vomiting or sit on the wound and transmit the pathogens.

Chapter 8

Cultivation of Bacteria

The laboratory culture of pathogenic microbes isolated from clinical specimens remains the backbone of laboratory diagnosis of infectious diseases. All the microbes cannot be grown in the laboratory and growth of the normal flora must be carefully eliminated, so that one can determine the causal agent for the ailment. Some specimens are normally sterile (*e.g.* blood, spinal fluid) while others, like feces are highly contaminated. Whenever possible, the preliminary report of the direct examination should be followed by a confirmatory report of the laboratory culture of the organisms. Special medium for growing the organism, culture conditions (*e.g.* aerobic, anaerobic, temperature *etc.*), colony characters, biochemical and other reactions are some of the features that help in the identification of the pathogenic microbe.

Culture Media

Artificial media, with known ingredients (glucose, protein, salt, vitamin, special chemicals) are used in the laboratory for the growing microbes. These media act as substrates for the pathogenic microorganisms. By adding increasing concentration of agar, consistency of the culture media can be varied-liquid, solid (20 per cent) or semisolid (0.5 per cent). Solid media are used for the isolation of colonies growing on the medium. Semisolid media are used for the testing motility. Media are placed in part dishes and test tubes for culturing microbes.

Simple Media

These media allow most organisms to grow and can be prepared as broth or as solid media. These are frequently used as a basic media to which other materials are added. Some of the most commonly used general purpose media include trypticase soy broth, trypticase soy agar, brain heart infusion broth or agar, blood agar and peptone water. Mueller Hinton agar is a general purpose medium that is specially used in the antibiotic sensitivity test.

Differential Media

These are capable of differentiating between two organisms by their characteristic reactions in the medium like haemolysis or biochemical changes. The haemolytic reaction on the blood agar plate differentiates beta haemolytic *Streptococcus pyogenes* or *Staphylococcus aureus* from alpha haemolytic *Streptococcus pnenmoniae*. Lactose fermenters (*e.g. Escherichia coli*) can be differentiated from non-lactose fermenters (*e.g. Shigella*) on McConkey lactose agar and EMB agar plates.

Selective and Selective-Differential Media

Selective media allow only a selective group of organisms to grow while inhibiting others. The inhibition is brought about by a number of inhibitors like bile salts, dyes, antibiotics and other. Some of the selective media play a dual role and can also differentiate various groups of organisms. This is often based on their biochemical reactions on the medium. These are called selective-differential media (*e.g.* McConkey, EMB).

Enrichment Media

Enrichment media are those, which favor the growth of one group organisms over another. This is specially used for the culture of fecal material intended for the laboratory identification of *Shigella* and *Salmonella*.

Three enrichment media are commonly used: GN broth, tetrathionate broth and selenite F broth. Selenite F broth can also serve as transportation media for the stool specimen Selenite broth is most effective under reduced oxygen tension. Therefore, it is dispensed in to tubes to a depth of 5 cm and inoculated heavily with fecal material.

Transport Media

Transport medium inhibits self-destruction of microorganisms. Thus the specimen maintains a "Status quo" condition. Delay during the transport of specimens from the point of collection noticeably affects the viability of delicate organisms and anaerobes. Various media are used for transporting different type of specimen *e.g.* Stuart transport medium is used for CSF and cervical specimens. This medium preserves *Neisseria* species and *Trichomonas* (for 24 hours). Cary-Blair and Amies transport media are used for transporting fecal material on rectal swabs, and are effective in preserving Salmonella.

Biochemical Test Media

Various pathogenic organisms have characteristic biochemical reactions in the media. This can be useful tool for their identification. The biochemical changes are recognized by the change in the color of the dye added to the medium or by the addition of external reagents *e.g.* triple sugar iron media, citrate media *etc.*

Aseptic Transfer of Microbes

Microbes are present everywhere, and hence it is necessary to use extreme care not to introduce unwanted organisms into container which holds the medium. The unwanted organisms may be introduced by direct contact with contaminated surfaces (hand, table, loop or needle) that have not been sterilized or through the air. Hence aseptic transfer that involves the transfer of microbes from one to another without contamination is important. Inoculating needle and loop are the basic implements used in the transfer of inoculum from the specimen to the medium or from one medium to another. The needle is made of straight wire, while the loop is a wire that has been rounded at the tip. The wire is usually platinum or an alloy, such as nitrochrome, that can be heated to glowing without being damaged, and returns to room temperature fairly rapidly. When a transfer is to be made the needle or loop is sterilized in a flame, perform the transfer, and then resterilized before it is set aside.

Various Method of Inoculation of Bacteria

Inoculation of Test Tubes

The test tubes may contain broth media or it may be an agar slant. While transferring the inoculum into a test tube, in general, the cotton plug or cap is removed with, and held in, the outer three fingers of the hand holding the inoculating needle. The lip of the tube is flamed before and after entry to prevent contamination of the culture. The transfer is performed with a sterilized inoculating loop.

1. Assemble the materials needed on the hand.
2. Hold the tube in your left hand.
3. Hold the inoculating loop in your right hand (for right hander) and sterilize by flaming. Cool the loop.
4. Pick up the inoculum with the sterilized loop.
5. Remove the cap or other closure by wrapping the little finger of your right hand around the cap of the tube nearest to your right hand. Grab only the upper most portion of the cap.
6. Transfer the inoculum to the medium if it is a broth. If it is an agar slant, inoculate the culture by gentle rubbing on the surface of the medium.
7. Re-flame the neck of the tube and recap it.

Transfer to Petri Dishes

Microorganisms are commonly grown in petri dished or test tubes. While transferring the inoculum on the surface of agar in a petri dish, the following method is recommended:

1. Sterilized the loop (or needle) on the flame.
2. Cool the loop in the air so that the hot needle does not cremate the living bacterial cells to be transferred.

3. Pick up the specimen (or colony) to be planted with the sterilized loop.
4. Open the lid half way with your hand and streak the plate. Do not expose the agar surface more than necessary. While flaming the loop during streaking keep the lid fully closed.

Bacterial cultures may be inoculated on the agar plates using various methods depending on the purpose of inoculation. They may be:

1. Spot Inoculation

Spot inoculation is done where the bacteria is required to grow in a specified area in the medium. This is mainly used to detect toxin production by the bacteria.

Procedure

1. Sterilize the inoculation loop and take small amount of bacterial culture.
2. Under aseptic conditions raise the lid of petridish and rub the loop at a particular spot on the agar surface.
3. Close the lid and incubate the plate.

2. Streaking or Streak Plate Method

Pure culture of the infectious agent is necessary for the correct identification of the pathogen. Streaking is one of the common methods of obtaining pure culture on the primary plate. In this process small amount of the specimen (called inoculum is spread out (called streaking) on a solid medium which leads to the development of mixed discrete colonies of inhabiting organisms in the specimen. An isolated colony can then be transferred to a secondary medium to obtain a pure culture.

Procedure

Prepare the solid agar plates in advance. The agar surface should be dry. The number of plates needed for the day should be kept at room temperature until the time of inoculation. Plating on a "chilled plate" is not recommended.

1. Place a small amount of inoculum near the periphery of the plate.
2. Spread the inoculum over a zone by to and fro movement of the loop.

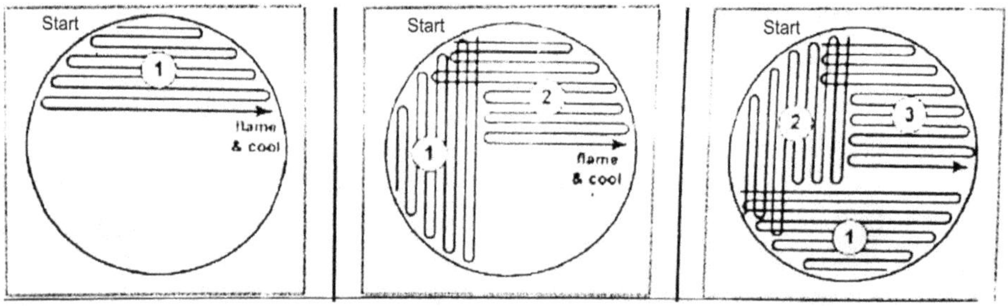

Streak area 1
Sterilized the loop

Rotate counterclockwise.
Spread area 1over area 2.
Sterilize the loop.

Rotate counterclockwise spread
area 2 over area 3.
Sterilize the loop.

Figure 8.1: Streaking or Streak Plate Method.

3. Turn the plate 45°, overlap the previous streak at several point and steak at 90° of the previous one.
4. Again turn the plate at 45° and repeat as previously.
5. Finally, lift the loop and streak the center of the plate with zigzag motion in the remaining part of the plate.

3. Pour Plate Method

Pour plate method is generally used for quantitation of bacteria in samples (like milk, meat, sweet, water *etc.*). After mixing a known amount of sample into molten agar medium the number of bacterial colonies is counted to get number of viable bacteria per unit of the sample.

Procedure

1. Prepare the nutrient agar, adjust pH and sterilize by autoclaving.
2. Allow the nutrient agar to cool at 45°C.
3. Add a known quantity (*e.g.* 0.1 ml) of the sample in the petridish and 15-20ml of molten agar as per the size of petridish.
4. Mix the sample with agar thoroughly by swirling motions.
5. Cover the petridish with lid and allow it to solidify.
6. Incubate at 37°C for 24-48 hrs.
7. Count the number of bacterial colonies appearing in the plate by the naked eye or with the help of colony counter.

Result

The total number of bacteria per ml of sample can be calculated by multiplying number of bacteria to the dilution factor.

3. Stab Culture Method

The stab inoculation is required for some specific purposes *e.g.* to study the biochemical reactions in Triple Sugar Iron medium.

Procedures

1. Prepare the medium adjust pH and sterilize by autoclaving.
2. Prepare the slants with a butt.
3. Unfold the inoculation loop to make it a straight needle.
4. Pick up a small amount of bacterial culture on the tip of straight needle.
5. Under aseptic conditions introduce the straight needle into the slant medium until it reaches to the bottom of the test tube. Withdraw the needle in the same path without breaking the medium and make a zigzag streak on the surface of slant before withdrawing the needle.
6. Plug the tube and incubate at 37°C for 24 to 48 hrs.

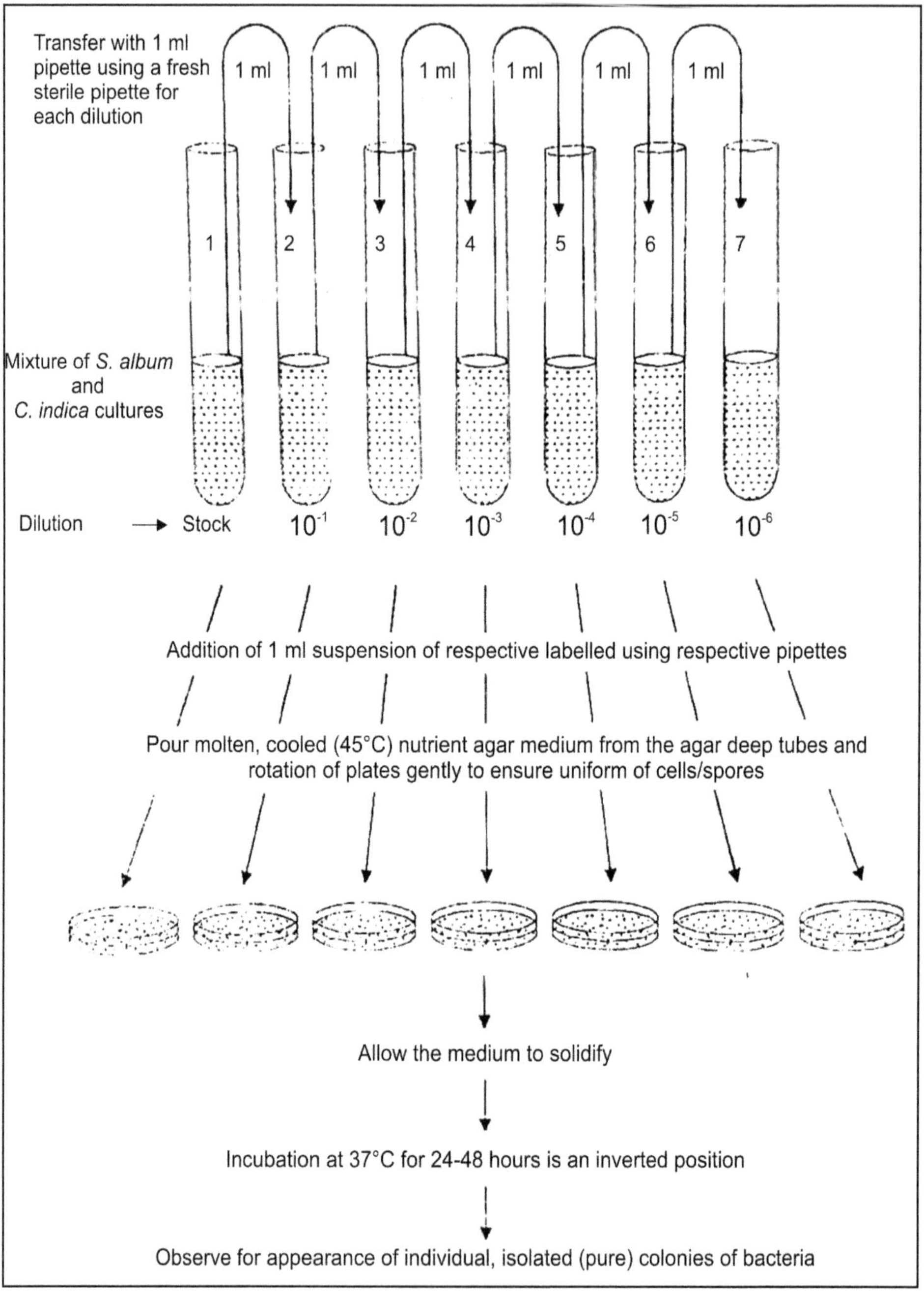

Figure 8.2: Pour Plate Method.

Bacterial Colony Characteristics

A bacterial colony is a very homogeneous population formed by the progeny of a single bacterium. The colony becomes visible with the naked eye after several millions of individual are produced. Since all the members of the colony are derived from a single cell, all the characteristics of the bacteria within that population are essentially the same. Different bacteria (*i.e.* different species, and sometimes strains) have specific colony characteristics on specific media. Thus, evaluation of colony characteristics is one of the first steps in the process of identifying bacteria. Always select a typical well isolated colony for your observations. Crowded colonies are going to be small due to competition for nutrients between adjacent colonies.

There are seven macroscopic characteristics of bacterial colonies that must be served and recorded. These are:

- **Size**: whenever possible measure colony diameter and express it in millimeters mm. If the bacteria colony is too small to be measured you may describe it as punctiform (*Pin point, small, moderate or large*)
- **Shape**: The shape of the colony.
  - Circular – Unbroken peripheral edge.
  - Irregular – Indented peripheral edge.
  - Filamentous – Thread like, spreading growth.
  - Spindle – Spindal shape colony.
  - Punctiform – Pin point colony
  - Rhizoid – Root like spreading growth.
- **Margin**: Describe the outer edge of the colony.
  - Entire – Sharply defined, even.
  - Undulate – Wavy indentations.
  - Filamentous – Thread like spreading edge.
  - Lobate – Marked indentations.
  - Serrate – Tooth like appearance (Erose)
  - Curled – Like curly degree to hairs with parallel filaments.
- **Surface**: select one of (a) and one from (b)
  a) smooth, wrinkled, rough, concentric rings
  b) dull (matte), or shiny (glistening)
- **Pigmentation**: Describe the color of the colony.
- **Transmited Light**: hold the plate up to the light. Call it translucent if the light passes through the colony or opaque if the light does not pass through the colony
- **Elevation**: The degree to which colony growth is raised on the agar surface.
  - Flat – Elevation not discernible.
  - Raised – Slight elevatiov.

- ❒ Convex – Dome shaped elevation.
- ❒ Umbonated - Raised with elevated convex, central region (Convex with a central knob).
- ❒ Pulvinate – Large dome shaped elevation.

☆ **Opacity** – opaque, translucent, transparent.

☆ **Consistanct** – Butyrous, friable, viscis (sticky).

☆ **Emulsification** – Easy, difficult, form homogenous or granular suspension.

Culture Characteristics of Bacteria

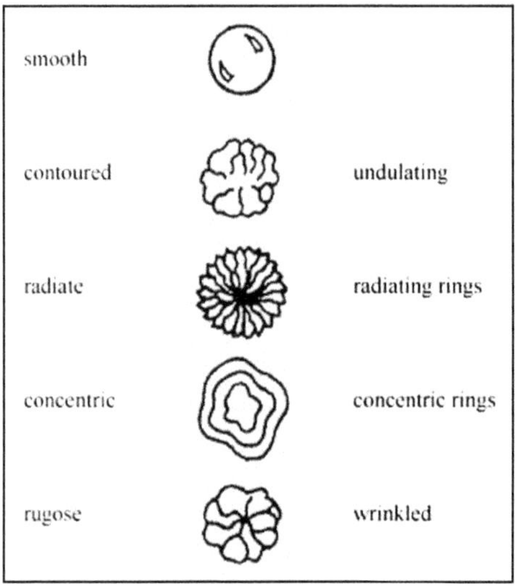

Colony Morphology: Surface of Colony.

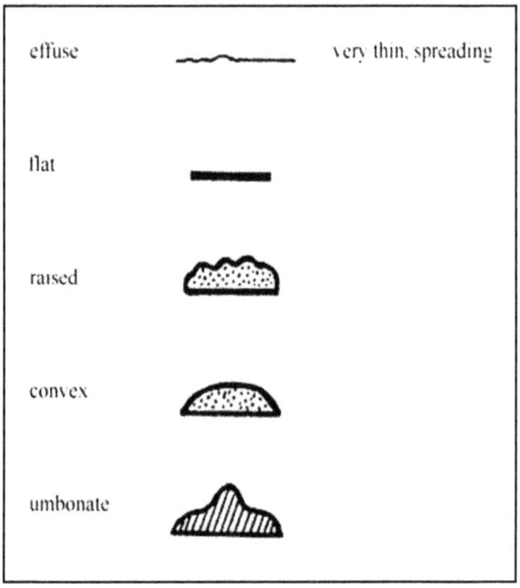

Colony Morphology: Elevation of colony.

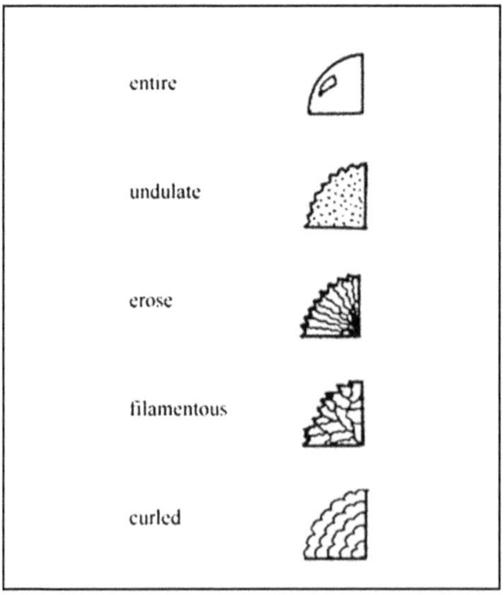

Colony Morphology: Margin of colony.

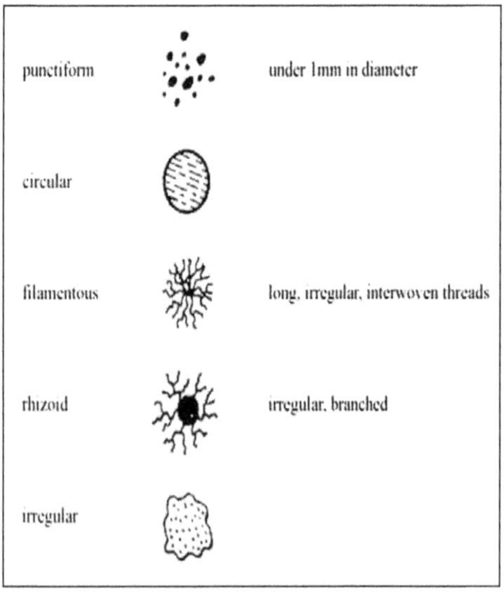

Colony Morphology: Form of colony.

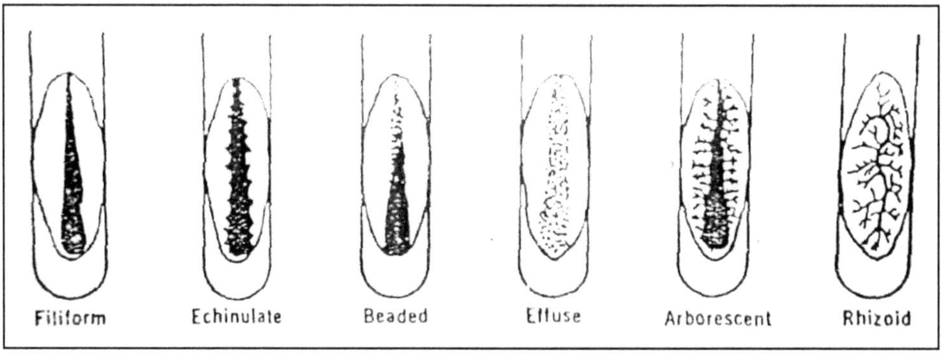

Figure 8.3: Form of Bacterial Growth on Agar Slant.

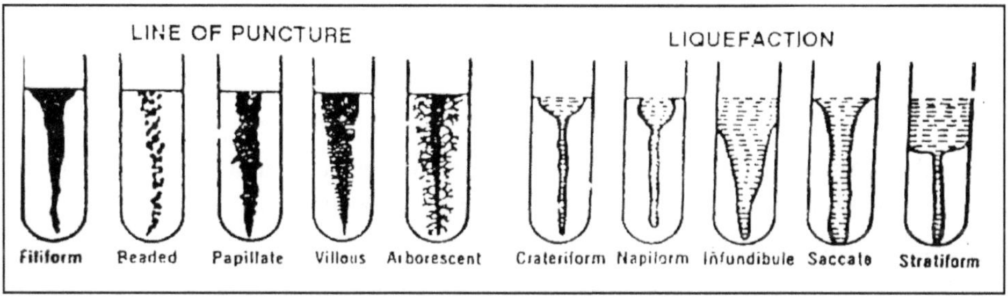

Figure 8.4: Form Liquefaction Pattern in Agar Stab.

Growth on Nutrient Agar Slant

They have a single straight line of inoculation on the surface and evaluated in the following manner.

I. Amount of growth – Abundance of growth is designated an none, scanty (slight), moderate or large, abundant.

II. Pigmentation – Chromogenic bacteria may produce intracellular pigments that are responsible for the colouration of the organism ae seen in surface colonies. Other organisms produce extra cellular soluble pigments that are excreted in the medium and also produce a colot. Most organisms, however, are non-chromogenic and will appear white to gray.

III. Consistency – May be evaluated on the basis of the amount of light transmitted through the growth. This is described as opaque (no light transmission), translucent (partial transmission) or transparent (full transmission).

IV. Form of growth – The appearance of the single line of streak of growth on the agar surface is designated as –

- ✰ Filiform – Characterized by uniform growth along the line of inoculation.
- ✰ Effuse – Growth is thin veil – like, unusually spreading.
- ✰ Echinulate – Margins of growth exhibit toohed appearance.

- ☆ Beaded – Separate or semiconfluent colonies along the line of inoculation.
- ☆ Arborescent – Branched, tree like growth.
- ☆ Rhizoid – Root – like appearance.

Nutrient Broth Cultures

These are evaluated to the distribution and appearance of the growth in the medium.

- ☆ Amont of growth – Scanty, moderate, abundant.
- ☆ Surface growth – Abscent and present
  - ❒ Ring like
  - ❒ Pellicle
  - ❒ Flocculent
  - ❒ Membranous
- ☆ Turbidity- Absent oe present (dispersed growth throughout)
- ☆ Sedimentation (Deposit) – Concentration of growth at the bottom of the broth culture, may be granular, flaky or flocculent.
- ☆ Odour – Present or absent

Anaerobic Cultivation of Bacteria

Respiration is an energy yielding process in which electrons from an oxidizable substrate are transferred via a series of oxidation – reduction reactions to an exogenous terminal electron transport chain. Microorganisms differ in their ability to use oxygens for cellular respiration. Some bacteria require an increased concentration of carbon dioxide in their environment. This concentration may vary from 3 to 10 per cent. One of the easy ways is to use the candle jar technique. If Brewer jar is used, the CO_2 concentration can be raised to 10 per cent. Anaerobic bacteria cannot cultivated in the presence of oxygen. Anaerobic bacteria can be cultivated by different methods.

A. Deep agar column method.
B. Roll tube method of Hungate
C. Alkali-pyrogallic acid method
D. Buchner's method
E. Wright's method
F. Anaerobic Jar method
   - ☆ McIntosh Jar Method
   - ☆ Brewer Jar Method

Modified McIntosh – Fildes Jar Method

The principle of the apparatus is that spongy palladium or spongy platinum acting as a catalytic agent causes the slow combination of hydrogen and oxygen to form water. The jar is made of stout glass or metal and has a tight fitting lid with rubber gasket. Lid can be clamped down. Rubber gasket eliminates the need for plasticene or grease. The catalyst, made of pellets of alumina coated with Pallidium and contained in a Monal metal gause envelope, is active at room temperature and dispenses with the need for electricity. Thus reducing the danger of explosion. The lid has two needle valves, one for attachment to vacuum and monometer and I for attachment to gas sources.

A. Candle Jar Technique

1. Take a glass container that holds several petri dishes and can be tightly sealed. If using a screw-capped jar, make sure that there is a rubber seal. If gas jars are used put grease on the rim so that glass plate fits airtight.
2. Place the inoculated plates in the jar in an inverted position (lid facing down).
3. Now affix a candle to the inside of a petri dish lid, and set it in the jar on top of the inoculated plates.
4. Light the candle and seal the jar tightly. The oxygen inside the jar will be used up by the burning candle and replaced by carbon dioxide, the candle will go out, and a 3 to 5 per cent carbon dioxide atmosphere will then be created. This suits the needs of microaerophiles.

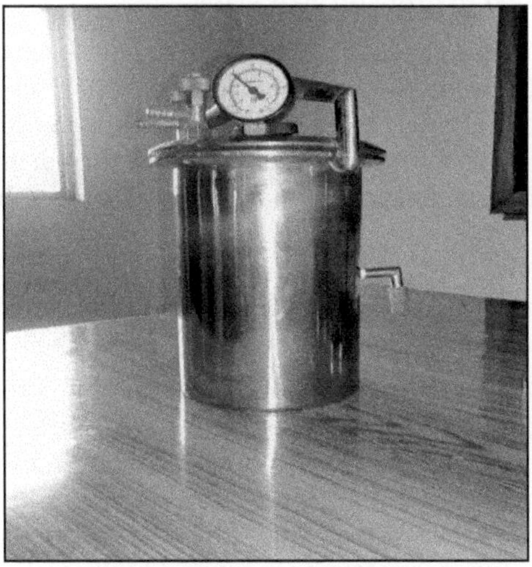

Figure 8.5: Anaerobic Jar.

Brewer Jar Method

A self- contained hydrogen carban dioxide anaerobic system was developed by Brewer and Allgeier. The system eliminates the need for gas cylinders, vacuum pumps, valves and gauses. It makes use of the standard pyrex glass anaerobic jar with a new anaerobic lid that is fitted with a snap- in rubber gasket, a double stainless steel gauze flash arrestor, and a catalyst holder that contains alumina pellets coated with 0.5 per cent palladium. This catalyst is active at room temperature and does not require heating. The system uses a disposable hydrogen carbon dioxide generator and a disposable methylene blue anaerobic indicator.

Procedure

1. Inoculate the slant and nutrient agar plate with anaerobic bacteria sample in front of flame.
2. Place the inoculated plates and tubes inside the jar.
3. Place and cut the corner of hydrogen carbon dioxide gaspak
4. Place disposable methylene blue indicator.
5. Add 10 ml water in gaspak with help of pipette.
6. The lid is clamped in place and the jar is placed in the incubator.
7. Methylene blue indicator gradually changes from blue to colorless as the oxygen in the jar is utilized this occurs within several hours.
8. Incubate the jar for for 24 to 48 hours, after incubation open the jar and examine the growth of anaerobic bacteria.

B. Alkaline Pyrogallol Method

In this method the reducing agent is kept in the empty space of culture tube and anaerobe is allowed to grow on agar slant.

This procedure helps in isolation of bacteria in pure form, which is not possible with the broth culture. The method is tricky and hence not too popular. It is adopted only when it is absolutely necessary. An anaerobic condition is established by activating pyrogallol with sodium carbonate, which then acts as a strong reducing agent and removes the free oxygen from a tightly stopper tube.

Procedure

1. Take a nutrient agar slant with a cotton plug and inoculate it with the anaerobic microorganisms to be tested. Label the tube.
2. Cut of the protruding portion of the cotton plug. Push the remaining half of the plug down into the tube with the handle of inoculation loop to within 1cm from the tip of the agar slant. The cotton plug must fit tightly so that the chemicals placed on it will not seep into the agar until you can invert the tube. At the same time, it must allow free passed of gases between the two compartments created by the cotton plug.
3. With a clean weighing spoon, add pyrogallol crystals to within about 2cm. of the neck of the tube.
4. Add one dropper full of 10 per cent sodium carbonate (aqueous solution) to the dry pyrogallol. Work as rapidly as possible from this point on to avoid seepage of these chemicals through the cotton onto the agar. Furthermore, the small amount of sodium carbonate and pyrogallol used can only reduce a limited amount of oxygen.

5. Place a rubber stopper in to the neck of the tube and simultaneously invert the tube and twist the rubber stopper until an airtight seal is formed.
6. To ensure tight seal, apply a strip of masking tape over the top of the rubber stopper and warp a second strip around the rubber stopper juncture several times.
7. Once the tube is inverted, keep it in the inverted position in a wire basket.
8. Incubated at 35°C for 24 to 48 hours or longer.

Chapter 9

Identification of Bacteria

There are two methods for the identification of bacteria.

1. Primary identification of bacteria
2. Secondary identification of bacteria

1. Primary Identification of Bacteria

Once a pure culture is obtained the results from a few comparatively simple tests can often identify the bacterium to a generic level.

I. *By microscopic examination-* This method is useful to determine the morphological appearance like shape, size, arrangement, motility and on the staining behavior.

II. *Cultural characteristic* – Colonies appearance are useful criteria for the identification of bacteria. Examples *Streptococcus pyogenes* produces pin head colonies with beta -haemolysis whereas *Staphylococcus albus* is without any haemolysis.

III. *By Chemical test*:

- ☆ Catalase test
- ☆ Oxidase test
- ☆ Oxidation/Fermentation (O/F) test
- ☆ Sugar fermentation

Catalase Test

Catalase is the name of an enzyme found in most bacteria, which initiates the breakdown of hydrogen peroxide (H_2O_2) into water and free oxygen. Most bacteria are catalase positive; however certain genera that do not carry out aerobic respiration, such as *Streptococcus, Lactobacillus* and *Clostridium* are catalase negative.

Procedure

Add a few drops of 3 per cent hydrogen peroxide to each culture and look for the release of oxygen as a result of hydrogen peroxide break down, alternatively, take few drops of 3 per cent hydrogen peroxide in a test tube and transfer bacterial colonies using a glass rod or a plastic loop.

"If the organism has catalase activity, foaming or effervescence will appear within 10-30 seconds".

Oxidase Test

This test depends on the presence of cytochrome C oxidae in a bacterial cell. Aerobes, facultative anaerobes and microaerophils posses this enzymes whill the anaerobes donot. Oxidase enzymes cytochrome oxidase catalyses the oxidation of reduced cytochrome by molecular oxygen resulting in the formation of water or H_2O_2. Oxidase enzyme in the presence of air, acts on certain aromatic amines to produce coloured compounds.

Procedure

A strip of filter paper is soaked in 1per cent aquas solution of the reagent N,N,N,N tetra methyl p-phenylene diamine dihydrochloride.

Culture is rubbed on the filter paper produces intense red color within 5-10 seconds in positive, if not then negative.

Oxidation/Fermentation (O/F) Test

This test is used to determine Oxidation/Fermentative metabolism of carbohydrate by the bacteria. In oxidation molecules oxygen serves as final electron acceptor while in fermentation on organic substrate serves as final electron acceptor.

Procedure

Take two test tubes of Hugh Leifson (H.L) medium and heat it before use, to remove the dissolved oxygen. Then cool it. Inoculate the culture by stab-inoculation technique, sealed the test tube and incubated at 37°C for 24 hours. Examination is done per day.

Before inoculation medium color is blue but this color is changed to yellow on acid production.

Sl.No.	*Open tube*	*Sealed tube*	*Example*	*Reaction*
1.	Yellow	blue	*Pseudomonas*	Oxidation
2.	Yellow	Yellow	*Aeromonas*	Fermentation
3.	blue	blue	*Bordetella*	Un-reactive

Sugar Fermentation

Most microorganisms obtain energy through bio-oxidation of a substrate, mostly a carbohydrate. Organisms use sugars (mono, di and trisaccharides) depending on their enzyme compliment either aerobically, anaerobically or by both pathways. The fermentative or oxidative attack on sugars produces acid detected by pH indicator; gas may also be produced along with acidic metabolites.

Procedure

One percent sugar peptone water broth is inoculated with cultures. The durham's tube is inverted in the test tube containing culture broth and incubate it for 37°C for 24 hours.

Observation is done by acid production with gas/acid production with no gas/No acid production.

2. Secondary Identification of Bacteria

Once the bacterium has been identified to a generic level, further tests can be carried out to identify the species.

Biochemical Characters

IMViC Reactions

IMViC reactions are a set of four useful reactions that are commonly employed in the identification of members of family *enterobacteriaceae*. The four reactions are: Indole test, Methyl Red test, Voges Proskauer test and Citrate utilization test. The letter "i" is only for rhyming purpose.

Indole Test

Principle

Some bacteria can produce indole from amino acid tryptophan using the enzyme typtophanase.

$$\text{Tryptophan} = \xrightarrow[H_2O]{\text{Tryptophanase}} \text{Indole} + \text{Pyuruvic Acid} + NH_3$$

Production of indole is detected using Ehrlich's reagent or Kovac's reagent. Indole reacts with the aldehyde in the reagent to give a red color. An alcoholic layer concentrates the red color as a ring at the top.

Procedure

Bacterium to be tested is inoculated in peptone water, which contains amino acid tryptophan and incubated overnight at 37°C. Following incubation few drops of Kovac's reagent are added. Kovac's reagent consists of para-dimethyl aminobenzaldehyde, isoamyl alcohol and con. HCl. Ehrlich's reagent is more sensitive in detecting indole production in anerobes and non-fermenters. Formation of a red or pink coloured ring at the top is taken as positive.

Example

Escherichia coli: Positive; *Klebsiella pneumoniae*: Negative

Methyl Red (MR) Test

Principle

This is to detect the ability of an organism to produce and maintain stable acid end products from glucose fermentation. Some bacteria produce large amounts of acids from glucose fermentation that they overcome the buffering action of the system. Methyl Red is a pH indicator, which remains red in color at a pH of 4.4 or less.

Procedure

the bacterium to be tested in inoculated into glucose phosphate broth, which contains glucose and a phosphate buffer and incubated at 37°C for 48 hours. Over the 48 hours the mixed-acid producing organism must produce sufficient acid to overcome the phosphate buffer and remain acid. The pH of the medium is tested by the addition of 5 drops of MR reagent. Development of red color is taken as positive. MR negative organism produces yellow color.

Example

Eschericihia coli: Positive; *Klebsiella pneumoniae*: Negative

Voges Proskauer (VP) Test

Principle: While MR test is useful in detecting mixed acid producers, VP test detects butylene glycol producers.

Glucose → Acetoin

Acetoin KOH....... Diacetyl + H_2O

Atmospheric O_2

Diacetyl + guanidine component of peptone alpha naphthol Pink colour

Acetyl-methyl carbinol (acetoin) is an intermediate in the production of butylene glycol. In these test two reagents, 40 per cent KOH and alpha-naphthol are added to test broth after incubation and exposed to atmospheric oxygen. If acetoin is present, it is oxidized in the presence of air and KOH to diacetyl. Diacetyl then reacts with guanidine components of peptone, in the presence of alphanaphthol to produce red color. Role of alpha-naphthol is that of a catalyst and a color intensifier.

Procedure

Bacterium to be tested is inoculated into glucose phosphate broth and incubated for at least 48 hours. 0.6 ml of alpha-naphthol is added to the test broth and shaken. 0.2 ml of 40 per cent KOH is added to the broth and shaken. The tube is allowed to stand for 15 minutes. Appearance of red color is taken as a positive test.

The negative tubes must be held for one hour, since maximum color development occurs within one hour after addition of reagents.

Examples

Escherichia coli: Negative; *Klebsiella pneumoniae*: Positive

Citrate Utilization Test

Principle

This test detects the ability of an organism to utilize citrate as the sole source of carbon and energy. Bacteria are inoculated on a medium containing sodium citrate and a pH indicator bromothymol blue. The medium also contains inorganic ammonium salts, which is utilized as sole source of nitrogen.

$$\text{Citrate} \rightarrow \text{Oxaloacetate} + \text{Acetate}$$

$$\text{Oxaloacetate} \rightarrow \text{Pyruvate} + CO_2$$

$$CO_2 + Na + H_2O \rightarrow Na_2CO_3$$

Utilization of citrate involves the enzyme citritase, which breaks down citrate to oxaloacetate and acetate. Oxaloacetate is further broken down to pyruvate and CO_2. Production of Na_2CO_3 as well as NH_3 from utilization of sodium citrate and ammonium salt respectively results in alkaline pH. This results in change of medium's color from green to blue.

Procedure

Bacterial colonies are picked up from a straight wire and inoculated into slope of Simmon's citrate agar and incubated overnight at 37°C. If the organism has the ability to utilize citrate, the medium changes its color from green to blue.

Examples

Escherichia coli: Negative; *Klebsiella pneumoniae*: Positive

Bacterium	*Indole*	*MR*	*VP*	*Citrate*
E. coli	+	+	–	–
K. pneumoniae	–	–	+	+

Nitrate Reductase Test

Principles

Reduction of nitrate is generally an anaerobic respiration in which an organism derives its oxygen from nitrate. Depending upon environmental conditions, the end products of this metabolic process are usually not further oxidized or assimilated into cellular metabolism, but are excreted into the surrounding medium. *Enterobacteriaceae* characteristically reduce nitrate to nitrite which reacts with sulfanilic acid and N, N-dimethylalpha- naphthylamine to produce a red color (Griess reaction). The formation of other end products (ammonia, nitrous oxide, hydroxylamine, *etc.*) is also possible; therefore, the addition of zinc dust is used to detect unreduced nitrate. The formation of nitrogen gas, an end product typical of certain organisms, is evidenced by displacement of the medium from the Durham tube by the gas produced.

Procedure

1. Inoculate nitrate broth with an isolate and incubate for 48 hours.
2. Add 10-15 drops each of sulfanilic acid and *N*, *N*-dimethyl-1-naphthylamine. If the bacterium produces nitrate reductase, the broth will turn a deep red within 5 minutes at this step.
3. If no color change is observed, then the result is inconclusive. Add a small amount of zinc to the broth. If the solution remains colorless, then both nitrate reductase and nitrite reductase are present. If the solution turns red, nitrate reductase is not present.

Triple Sugar Iron Agar

Principles

TSI Agar contains three sugars (dextrose, lactose and sucrose), phenol red for detecting carbohydrate fermentation and ferrous ammonium sulfate for detection of hydrogen sulfide production (indicated by blackening in the butt of the tube). Carbohydrate fermentation is indicated by the production of gas and a change in the color of the pH indicator from red to yellow. To facilitate the detection of organisms that only ferment dextrose, the dextrose concentration is one-tenth the concentration of lactose or sucrose. The small amount of acid produced in the slant of the tube during dextrose fermentation oxidizes rapidly, causing the medium to remain red or revert to an alkaline pH. In contrast, the acid reaction (yellow) is maintained in the butt of the tube because it is under lower oxygen tension. After depletion of the limited dextrose, organisms able to do so will begin to utilize the lactose or sucrose. To enhance the alkaline condition of the slant, free exchange of air must be permitted by closing the tube cap loosely. If the tube is tightly closed, an acid reaction (caused solely by dextrose fermentation) will also involve the slant.

Procedure

To inoculate, carefully touch only the center of an isolated colony on an enteric plated medium with a cool, sterile needle, stab into the medium in the butt of the tube, and then streak back and forth along the surface of the slant. Several colonies from each primary plate should be studied separately, since mixed infections may occur. Incubate with caps loosened at 35°C and examine after 18-24 hours for carbohydrate fermentation, gas production and hydrogen sulfide production. Any combination of these reactions may be observed. Do not incubate longer than 24 hours because the acid reaction in the slant of lactose and sucrose fermenters may revert to an alkaline reaction.

Chapter 10

Bacterial Genetics

Introduction

The genetics of the bacteria from the basis of molecular biology. The objective is to know the variation that occurs in different bacteria.

Genetics

Genetics is the study of heredity and variation. It includes what are genes and how carry information from parents to their progeny and how to express the information within an organism determine the particular characteristics.

Chromosomes

Chromosomes are the cellular structures that physically carry hereditary information. They carry genes. They are single molecules of DNA arranged as double helix, in a closed loop.

Genes

Genes are located in circular chromosomes of bacteria and they are segments of DNA. Gene is the small unit of DNA.

Deoxyribonucleic Acid (DNA)

DNA is the store house of all genetic material and all informations for protein synthesis. DNA is made up of nucleotide (four nucleotide are Adenine (A), Thymine (T), Cystocine (C) and Guanine (G)). There are base of purine (A and G) and pyrimidine (C and T). There is backbone of alternating deoxyribose and phosphate, while purine and pyrimidine attached to sugar.

When a gene is expressed, DNA is transcribed to produce m-RNA, which is then translated to proteins. The DNA (in cells) is duplicated before cell division, sothat each daughter cell receives the same genetic information.

The bacteria are also containing RNA (Ribonucleic acid), which is structurally similar to DNA.

There is two basic differences one is ribose sugar in place of deoxyribose and other is one pyrimidine base is uracil in place of thymine in DNA.

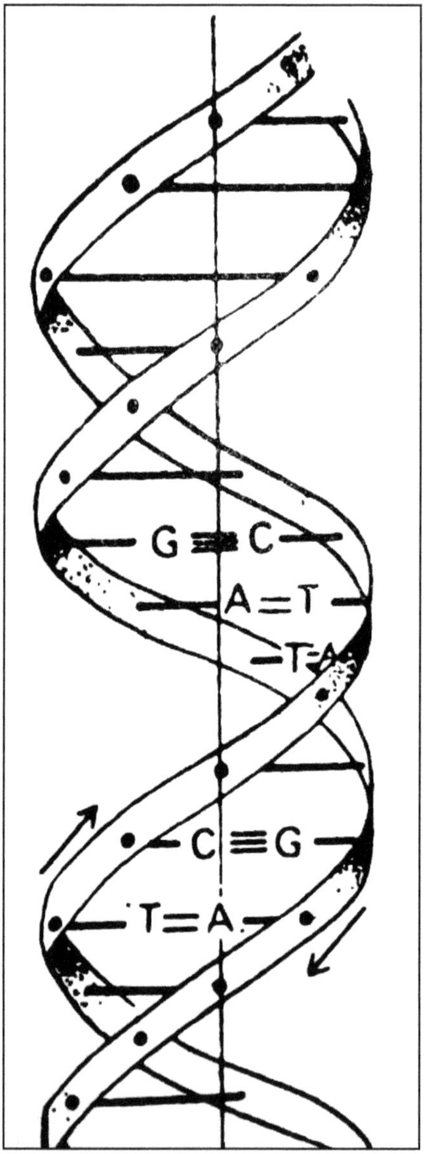

Figure 10.1: DNA Double Helix.

Deoxyribonucleic Acid (DNA)

Bacteria having a single circular chromosomes consisting of a single circular molecules of DNA.

In DNA replication, one parental double strand DNA is converted to identical daughter molicules. The two strand of the double standard helix separate at replication fork and each strand are used as template by DNA polymerase to synthesize two new strands of DNA. As the replication fork moves along with the parental DNA, each of the unwound single strands combines with the new nucleotides. The parental strand and newly synthesized daughter strand then rewind. Each new double strand contains one parental and one new strand. Replication fork meets when replication is completed.

The DNA of cell replicates before cell division so that each daughter cell receive an identical parental's chromosome. Genetic information contained in the DNA also flows in another ways. It is transcribed into mRNA and translated to proteins. DNA replication is an accurate process because of the proof reading capacity of DNA polymerase as it allows only correct complementary base to pairing structure.

At the replication fork, many replication enzymes assemble on the DNA into a complex molecular machine called the replisome. The following is a list of major DNA replication enzymes that participate in the replisome.

Table 10.1: DNA Replication Proteins

Enzyme	*Function in DNA Replication*
DNA Helicase	Also called helix destabilizing enzyme. Helicase separates the two strands of DNA at the replication fork behind the topoisomerase.
DNA Polymerase	The enzyme responsible for catalyzing the addition of nucleotides substrates to DNA in the 5^{I} to 3^{I} direction during DNA replication.
DNA clamp	A protein which prevents elongating DNA polymerases from dissociating from the DNA parent strand.
Single stranded binding proteins	Bind to ss DNA and prevents the DNA double helix from re-annealing after DNA helicase unwindsits, thus maintain the strand separation and facilitating the synthesis of the nascent strand.
Topoisomerase	Relaxes the DNA from its super –coiled nature.
DNA gyrase	Relieves strain of unwinding by DNA helicase, this is a specific type of topoisomerase.
DNA Ligase	Re-anneals the semi-conservative strands and join okazaki fragments of the lagging strand.
Primase	Provide a starting point of RNA (or DNA) for DNA polymerase to begine synthesis of the new DNA strand.
Telomerase	Lengthens telomeric DNA by adding repetitive nucleotide sequences to the ends of eukaryotic chromosomes. This allows germ cells and stem cells to avoid the Hayflick limit on cell division.

Proteins Synthesis

Transcription

It is synthesis of complementary strand of RNA called messenger RNA (mRNA) from a DNA. The mRNA carries the coded information for making specific proteins from DNA to ribosome where proteins are synthesized.

Ribosomal RNA (r-RNA)

Which forms integral part of ribosome, the cellular machinery for protein synthesis.

Transfer RNA (t-RNA)

Involved in protein synthesis, which carry amino-acid in a activated form to ribosome for the peptide bond formation in a sequence determined by m-RNA. If the template portion of DNA has a base sequence of ATGCAT, the newly synthesized strands have base sequence UACGUA.

Stepwise

1) RNA polymerase bind to DNA at a site known as promoter, double strand DNA, one strand act as template for RNA synthesis.

↓

2) RNA polymerase assembled free nucleotides into the chain, using complementary base pairing.

↓

3) New chain (RNA) grows and RNA polymerase moves with DNA.

↓

4) RNA synthesis continues until the RNA polymerase reaches to the terminal end of DNA.

↓

5) At this stage RNA polymerase and newly formed single strand m-RNA are released from the DNA.

RNA Splicing

Most of the genes in higher eukaryotes like birds and mammals are discontinuous and are split. The coding sequences of split genes are called **exons** whereas untranslated intervening sequences are called interons. Interons are sequences that are split out in the formation of mature RNA molecules process is called RNA splicing.

* The pre-messenger RNA thus formed contains introns, which are not required for protein synthesis. The pre-messenger RNA is chopped upto remove the introns and creates messenger RNA (mRNA).

Alternative Splicing

In this, individual exons are either spliced or included, giving rise to several different possible mRNA products. Each m-RNA product codes for a different protein isoform, these protein isoform differs in their peptides sequence and therefore their biological activity.

Alternative splicing contributes to protein diversity a single gene transcript (RNA) can have thousand s of different splicing patterns and will code for thousands of different proteins. A diverse proteome is generated from a limited genome. Splicing is important in genetic regulation abnormal splicing leads to disease development like cancer.

Translation

It is the process in which the m-RNA determines the amino-acid sequence of the protein. The m-RNA is in the form of codons, group of three nucleotides, such as AUG, GGC or AAA. The sequence of the codon on an m-RNA will determine the sequence of amino acid that synthesized proteins. Each codon 'code' for a particular amino-acid and this is called genetic code.

Table 10.2: Genetic Code – Triplet Codon Assignments for the 20 Amino Acids

First Base (5' end)	*Middle Base*	*Third Base (3' end)*			
		U	*C*	*A*	*G*
U	U	Phe	Phe	Leu	Leu
	C	Ser	Ser	Ser	Ser
	A	Tyr	Tyr	Stop	Stop
	G	Cys	Cys	Stop	Tri
C	U	Leu	Leu	Leu	Leu
	C	Pro	Pro	Pro	Pro
	A	His	His	Gln	Gln
	G	Arg	Arg	Arg	Arg
A	U	Lle	Lle	Lle	Met
	C	Thr	Thr	Thr	Thr
	A	Asn	Asn	Lys	Lys
	G	Ser	Ser	Arg	Arg
G	U	Val	Val	Val	Val
	C	Ala	Ala	Ala	Ala
	A	Asp	Asp	Glu	Glu
	G	Gly	Gly	Gly	Gly

Genetic Code

The genetic code is universal. It is the basis of the transmission of hereditary information by nucleic acid in all organisms. There are four bases in RNA (A, G, C and U), there are 64 triplet codes (4^3=64) but only 20 amino-acids with additional to start and stop codon. Many amino-acid have several codes (degeneracy) so that all 64 triplet codes are used. Out of 64 codons, 61 are sense codons and rest three are non-sense codons (also known as stop codon). The non-sense codons (UAA, UAG and UGA) signal the end of protein synthesis. Start codon AUG, that initiate the protein synthesis, which is also the codon for methionine. The methionine is often removed later, so not all proteins begin with methionine. The codons of m-RNA are converted into protein by the process of translation. The amino-acid is brought by the t-RNA and assembled into a chain, at the site of translation that is ribosome.

Function of Ribosomes

Ribosomes are that direct order, binding of t-RNA to codon and to assemble the amino-acid into a growing chain so that producing a protein.

Note: Each amino-acid has its own special t-RNA.

Exp. T-RNA for phenylalanine (t-RNA Phe) is different from the histidine (t-RNA His). Each amino-acid is attached to its t-RNA through the 3'OH' group to form an ester, which react with the alph-amino group of the terminal amino-acid of the growing protein chain to form a new amide bond (peptide bond) during protein synthesis. The reaction of esters with amines is generally favourable but the rate of reaction is increased greatly in the ribosome.

Flow-chart

The two ribosomal subunit and the m-RNA molecules to be translated, along with several additional protein factors. This sets up the start codon (AUG) is allow translation process.

↓

First t-RNA to bind to the start codon, bring with it the amino-acid (methionine).

↓

t-RNA, recognizes the second codon, moves into position on the ribosome, the first amino-acid is transferred by the ribosome.

↓

Ribosome joins the two amino-acids with peptide bond, the first t-RNA molicules leaves the ribosome.

↓

Ribosome then move along with the m-RNA to the next codon.

↓

t-RNA bring the different amino-acid one by one and make a chain.

↓

Translation stops when m-RNA is reached to stop codon.

When the ribosomes reached at this codon. It comes apart into two subunits and m-RNA and the newly formed peptide chain are released. The ribosomes, m-RNA and t-RNA are then again available for further use.

Mutation

A mutation is the change in the base sequence of DNA. The change in the base sequence of DNA will cause a change in the product encoded by that gene. Mutation is a heritable variation and are irreversible. This is occur due to any defect or alteration in the process of transcription and production of miscoded m-RNA followed by alteration in the amino-acid sequence of the protein, that is the gene product. Mutation is a natural event, taking place all the time at its particular frequency in all the dividing form of life. Many mutations are never detected called silent mutation. Mutation is best appreciated when it involves a function which can be readily observed. For example, *E. coli* mutation that loses its ability to ferment lactose can be readily detected on Mac-Conkey agar but not on nutrient agar.

Types of Mutation

Mutations are the following types:

1) Frameshift Mutation

It is a mutation caused by insertion or deletion of a number of nucleotides that is not evenly divisible three from a DNA sequence. Also termed as *in-frame mutation.*

2) Non-sense Mutation

It is point mutation in a sequence of DNA that result in premature stop codon, or a non-sense codon in the transcribed m-RNA, and possibly a truncated and often non functional protein product.

3) Missense Mutation or Nonsynonymous Mutation

It is also point mutation, where single nucleotide is change to caused substitution of different amino-acid. This in turn can render the resulting protein nonfunctional.

4) Neutral Mutation

Neutral mutation is a mutation that occurs in amino-acid codon that results in the use of a different, but chemically similar, amino-acid. The similarity between the two is enough that little or no change is often rendered in the protein.

5) Silent Mutation

Silent mutations are mutations that do not result in a change to the amino-acid sequence of a protein, unless the changed amino-acid is sufficiently similar to the original. They may occur within a codon in a region that does not code for a protein, or they may occur within a codon in a manner that does not alter the final amino-acid sequence.

Mutagens

Chemical and radiation, which directly or indirectly bring mutation, are called mutagens. Almost any agents that chemically or physically react with DNA can cause mutations. Carcinogens are also mutagens that cause cancer in animal and man. The X-ray, U.V. rays and gamma rays, these are mutagenic. X-rays and gamma rays can cause ionization of DNA molecules resulting in error in DNA replication. The UV light, a non-ionizing component of sun light, can affect DNA by causing the formation of harmful covalent bonds between certain bases. Thymines in a DNA strand can cross link to form thymine dimmers, which can serious damage to the cell DNA.

Transmission of Genetic Material (Gene Transfer)

Genetic Recombination

Transfer of genetic material in bacteria occur as a result of transformation, transduction and conjugation. Recombination is determined by special genes (rec-genes).

Transformation in Bacteria

The process of transferring genetic characters from the donor to the receipient through the agency of small unit of DNA containing 10-15 genes. It was the first examples of genetic exchange in bacteria to have been discovered. Frederick Griffith in 1928 found that mice died when injected a mixture of live non-capsulated (R) pneumococci and heat killed capsulated (S) pneumococci, working on two strains of Streptococcus pneumonia,one is virulent strain, capsulated and other is a virulent strain non-capsulated. Griffith found that hereditary material from the dead bacteria had entered in living cells and there is genetically change and their progeny was encapsulated and virulent. This occurs due to transformation of genetic material, mechanism is told by O. Avery, C. MacLeod and M. Mc Carty in 1944.

In nature, when bacteria was die due to cell lysis, their DNA released into the environment, Other bacteria can encounter the DNA and depends on the species and growth condition, take up fragments of DNA and integrate them into their own chromosomes by recombination.

Conjugation in Bacteria

It is process by which donor bacterium make contact with recipient bacterium and transfer genetic material through sexual process. One type of genetic donor cell is an F^+, recipient is F^- cells. F^+ cell contain plasmids called F (fertility) factors; these are transferred to F^- cells during conjugation. In some cell carrying F factor, the factor integrates into the chromosome, converting the F^+ cell into Hfr cell (high frequency of recombination). During conjugation Hfr cell can transfer chromosomal DNA to an F^- cells. Hfr chromosome breaks before it is fully transferred.

In this process not the whole nucleoid but only definite parts of the nucleoid are transferred and this process takes place around 60 to 90 minutes

e.g. Conjugation can occur between *E. coli, Salmonella* and *Shigella etc.* in which antibiotics resistant gene (R factors) can be transferred. Conjugation has been occurring in various genera of bacteria called intergenic transfer.

Transduction

A portion of DNA is transfer from one bacterium to another with the help of bacteriophage is known as transduction. Transduction mechanism consisting following steps. During the multiplication of certain bacteriophages particularly the temperature phages they carry the genetic material of the bacterium and genetic material of the bacterium also enter into newly formed phage. When this newly formed phage, infect another bacterium the genetic material of the donor bacterium may recombine with the recipient bacterium and many hereditary characters are transduced.

Types

I) General transduction

II) Specific transduction

III) Abortive transduction

I) General Transduction

Recombination of genetic material carrying one or several charectors may occur.

II) Specific Transduction

Specific bacteriophage transduces only a particular genetic trait/specific characters can be transferred *e.g.* Galactose positive character.

III) Abortive Transduction

Characterized by the fact that genetic material carried by the phage is not incorporated into the genome of the recipient bacteria but remain in the cytoplasm of the bacteria and during cell division of the recipient bacterium the genetic material of the donor bacterium is transferred to one progeny cell. In abortive transduction is encountered ten times more frequently than the above two.

Extra Chromosomal Genetic Elements/Plasmid

Most bacteria possess extra chromosomal genetic elements that is not essential for normal life and functioning of host bacterium but may confer on it properties like druge resistance and toxigenicity leading to survival advantage under appropriate conditions.

Plasmids are circular DNA molecules present in the cytoplasm of bacteria, self-replicating, their ability to transfer genes from one cell to another. Plasmid is a important vector in genetic engineering. Plasmid may also found in yeast.

Plasmid DNA replicates in same ways as chromosomal DNA. Multiple copies of each plasmid may be present in a bacterial cell, although the number of copies depends upon the type of bacteria. The important properties carried by the plasmid are F (fertility) or F-plasmid, drug resistance factor (R-plasmid) and enterotoxigenic factors *etc.* These factors can be transferred from the donor to the recipient bacteria by the process transduction and conjugation.

Plasmid has been classified in different ways:

- ✰ Self transmissible or non transmissible
- ✰ On the property encoded like sex, drug resistance
- ✰ By restriction endonuclease finger printing
- ✰ By incompatibility typing

Closely related plasmids, do not coexist stably in the same bacterial cell,while unrelated plasmid can on this basis.

Transposons/Jumping Genes

A small segments of DNA that can move from one region to another region of the same chromosome or in different chromosomes or in a plasmid called transposons or jumping genes. Transposons are not self-replicating and depend on chromosomal or plasmid DNA for replication.

Chapter 11

Antibiotic Resistance

Introduction

The term antibiotic was first introduced by Salmon Waksman in 1941. The antibiotics are low molecular weight microorganisms metabolites that can have the ability or capacity to inhibit or kills the microbial growth.

Alexander flaming in 1929, first time recorded the antibiotic activity. He observed the lytic effect of the mould colony (*Penicillium notatum*) on neighbouring *Staphyloccocal* colonies on culture plate. Later on many antibiotics discovered and develop in pure form as in Table 11.1.

Antibiotic are specific products of metabolism or their modification with high physiological activity against individual group of microorganisms that kill or inhibit their growth. Antibiotics are a heterogeneous group of biologically active molecules with different structures and mode of action.

Mode of Action

Antibiotics are two types, bacteriostatic and bacteriocidal.

- ☆ **Bacteriostatic** – Antibiotics, which check or inhibit the bacterial growth.
- ☆ **Bacteriocidal** - Antibiotics, which kill the bacterial growth or population.

The growth of bacteria is also depends upon the host immune system, which eliminate the infection. Antibiotics may inhibit cell wall synthesis, effect on cell membrane function, inhibit protein synthesis and also inhibit the nucleic acid synthesis.

Table 11.1: Commonly Used Antibiotics, their Source and their Mode of Action

Antibiotics	*Source*	*Action*
Penicilline	*Penicillin notatum*	☆ Inhibit the cell wall synthesis. ☆ Mostly effective against gram positive.
Streptomycine	*Streptomyces griseus*	☆ Mostly effective against gram positive and gram negative. ☆ Interfered in protein synthesis.
Chloramphenicol	*Streptomyces venezuelae*	☆ Mostly effective against gram positive and gram negative. ☆ Inhibit in protein synthesis.
Lincomycin	*Streptomyces lincolensis*	☆ Mostly effective against gram positive and gram negative. ☆ Interfered in protein synthesis bind with 50s-ribosomal subunit.
Erythromycin	*Streptomyces erythreus*	☆ Mostly effective against gram positive and gram negative. ☆ Interfered in protein synthesis bind with 50s-ribosomal subunit.
Polymixin	*Bacillus polymyxa*	☆ Mostly effective against gram positive and gram negative. ☆ Rupture the cytoplsmic membrane
Bacitracin	*Bacillus licheniformis*	☆ Mostly effective against gram positive and gram negative. ☆ Interfered in protein synthesis bind with 50s-ribosomal subunit.
Oxytetracycline	*Streptomyces rimosus*	☆ Interfered in protein synthesis bind with 30s-ribosomal subunit. ☆ Inhibit in protein synthesis
Gentamicin	*Micromonospora* species	☆ Mostly effective against gram positive and gram negative. ☆ Inhibit in protein synthesis.
Vancomicin	*Streptomyces orientalis*	☆ Mostly effective against gram positive and gram negative. ☆ Inhibit in cell wall synthesis and interfere RNA synthesis.
Cephalosporin	*Cephalosporium* species	☆ Mostly effective against gram positive and gram negative. ☆ Inhibit in protein synthesis.

1) Inhibition of Cell Wall Synthesis

Bacterial cell wall

↓

Cell wall = made up of peptidoglycan layer

↓

Peptidoglycan layer = Made up of NAG and NAM

↓

Cross linking inhibited by antimicrobial agents

↓

Cell wall damaged

↓

Death of bacteria

For example-penicillins, cephalosporins and vancomycin antibiotics inhibit cell wall synthesis. If incorporating in the basic molecules of penicillin, it influences the antibiotic activity, stability and resistance to β-lactamases.

β-lactam antibiotics bind to cell receptors called as penicillin binding protein (PBPs). Such types of drugs increase autolysin activity resulting cell lysis. β-lactamases producing bacteria are resistant to β-lactam antibiotics by cleave the β-lactam ring in which becomes uneffective (inability to induce autolysin activity).

2) Inhibition of Cell Membrane Function

If any alteration in the cell membrane functions resulting macromolecules and ions escape from the cell leading to cell damage and death. Some of bactericidal antibiotics act on to damage the cell membrane. Such types of antibiotics are more toxic comparison to other.

3) Inhibition of Protein Synthesis or Faulty Protein Synthesis

- ☆ Causing faulty protein synthesis by binding to the 30 S ribosomal subunit for example amino-glycosides and tetracyclines.
- ☆ Causing faulty protein synthesis by binding to the 50 S ribosomal subunit for example Macrolides (erythromycin, azithromycin), lincosamide (Lincomycin, clindamycin) and chloramphenicol.

4) Inhibiting Bacterial Nucleic Acid Synthesis

- ☆ Inhibit DNA replication by inhibiting one or more of a group of enzymes called topoisomerases that are essential for bacterial DNA replication and transcription, for example quinolones (nor floxacine, ciprofloxacin).

- ☆ Inhibiting bacterial DNA synthesis by blocking synthesis of tetrahydrofolate, a cofactor needed to make nucleotide bases. Examples sulphonamide and trimethoprim.
- ☆ Drugs that are activated by the microbial proteins flavodoxin and feredoxin found in microaerophilic and anaerobic bacteria and certain protozoans. Once activated, the drug put nicks in the microbial DNA strands, such as metronidazole.

5) Multiple Actions

Blocks aerobic energy production and synthesis of proteins, DNA, RNA and cell wall. Example - nitrofurantoin.

Resistance of Bacteria to Antimicrobials

Most of the microbial resistance which is now making difficult to treat some infectious disease is of genetic origin and transferable between species and genera of bacteria. This is occurring due to extensive use of antimicrobial drugs, which favored the resistant strains of emerging disease. The excessive use and misuse of antimicrobials have lead to the death of sensitive strains leaving resistant strains to survive, multiply and infect new hosts.

Mechanisms of Antimicrobial Resistance

Some of the ways bacteria overcome the action of antimicrobials are as follows:

I) Due to genetic mutation, there is change in the bacterial cell component and proteins in which antimicrobial drugs are bind.

II) By producing enzymes that inactivate or destroy the antimicrobials.

III) By change in the cell membrane permeability, which make it difficult for entry of antimicrobials.

How to prevent the development of bacterial resistance

Following ways:

I) Reducing prophylactic use of antibiotics.

II) Increasing the therapeutic dose of antibiotics.

III) Use the antibiotics with the combination with other preparations.

Antibiotic Sensitivity Test

Most Pathogenic bacteria are susceptible to antibiotics or other antimicrobial agents but their response varies enormously. The antimicrobial susceptibility test provides help to the clinician to find out most effective antibiotic. The susceptibility test becomes necessary when the usually effective agents fail to produce desired effect and is mandatory in complex infectious syndromes. It requires 18 to 24 hrs to provide report to clinician.

Disc Diffusion Method

It is the most commonly used method for determination of antibiotic susceptibility Discs impregnated with known concentration of antibiotic are placed on an agar plate that has been inoculated or seeded uniformly over the entire plate with a culture of bacteria to be tested. The plate is incubated for 18 to 24 hrs at 37oc. During this period, the antimicobial agent diffuses through the agar and may prevent the growth of the organism. The effectiveness or susceptibility is proportional to the diameter of the inhibition zone around the disc. The organisms, which are grown up to the edge of the disc, are resistant.

Factors Affecting the Size of the Zone of Inhibition

The factors that can influence the size of the zone of inhibition are:

The Size of the Inoculums

The turbidity of the inoculums should be adjusted to 0.5 McFarland opacity standards. The aim is to have a dense lawn of bacterial growth with the individual colonies just touching each other. Failure to standardize the inoculums is a common source of error. Excess inoculums reduces the size of the inhibition zones whereas lesser inoculums not only make zone diameters difficult to read, but may fail to reveal resistance.

The inoculums are prepared from material picked up with a loop from five to ten colonies of the species to be tested. This material should be suspended in saline or broth, or grown as an overnight culture in broth. The suspension or culture should then be diluted to yield the correct weight of inoculums.

Turbidity Standard

It is prepared by pouring 0.6 ml of a 1 per cent (10 gm/L) solution of barium chloride dehydrate into a 100ml graduated cylinder and filling to 100 ml with 1 per cent (10 gm/L) sulphuric acid. The turbidy standard solution should be placed in a tube identical to the one use3d for the broth samples. It can be stored in the dark room temperature for six months, provided it is sealed to prevent evaporation.

The Test Medium

Muller- Hinton agar or its modification is usually chosen for routine susceptibility test, most pathogens grow satisfactory on the medium. For bacteria, such as *Streptococci*, that are unable to grow on Muller- Hinton agar with 5-10 per cent defibrinated sheep blood can be added. Chalgren agar is recommended for testing anaerobes. The pH of the medium must be close to 7.3. The depth of the agar must be 4mm (25 ml medium) in a flat-bottom 9cm diameter petri dishi on a level surface.

The Antimicrobial Agent and its Concentration on Disc

Commercially prepared sterile discs 6mm in diameter are used. Manufactures produce disc with accurate antibiotics content as recommended by WHO. The concentration of the antimicrobial agents in the discs have been chosen to give zone sizes that correlate with achievable serum levels in the patient.

The drug to be tested against each species of bacteria should be grouped in sets of six on a single 9cm diameter plate. The antibiotics in each set should be those most likely to be used for therapy of infections with a particular species. It is convenient to test routinely those antibiotics that are commonly prescribed by local clinicians (First line tests) and to reserve for later (Second line tests) those antibiotics for which prescription is restricted to special circumstances. Frequently, only one representative needs to be tests from any groups amongst which there is cross-resistance.

Incubation Conditions

These have been standardized for routine susceptibility tests under aerobic incubation at 35°C–37°C for 16-18 hours for the Staphylococci. The plates must not be incubated under an increased concentration of carban dioxide as this can significantly after the zones of inhibition with some antimicrobials agents. Plates should not be stacked more than three high (higher stacking could affect zone sizes).

The Test Bacterium

The degree of resistanmce or susceptibility of a bacterium to selected antimicrobial agents will vary with the species and strain of the pathogen.

Swabs

A supply of cotton wool swabs on wooden applicator sticks should be prepared. These can be sterilized in tins, culture tubes or on paper, either in the autoclave or by dry heat.

Procedures

1. Select the bacteria and prepare broth culture by inoculating into nutrient broth and incubating at 37°C for 24 hrs.
2. Prepare the Muller Hinton agar plates and test for sterility.
3. Take a sterilized swab and dip it into the inoculum and rotate firmly against the upper inside wall of the test tube to remove the fluid.
4. Streak (rub) the entire agar surface gently three times, turning the plate at 60°C between the streaks.
5. Replace the tops of plates and hold the plates at room temperature for about 5 min but not more than 15 min.
6. Place the commercially available antibiotic dishes, with the help of fine pointed pair of forceps, on to the agar surface. The centers of disc must be at least 24 cm apart.
7. After placing the disc on the agar surface, slightly press them with a sterile needle or forceps to make complete contact with surface of agar.

8. Incubate the test plates overnight at 37°C under appropriate condition suitable for the organisms.
9. Examine the plates after 18 to 24 hrs and later if necessary and measure the diameter of zone of inhibition of growth (including the diameter of the disc).

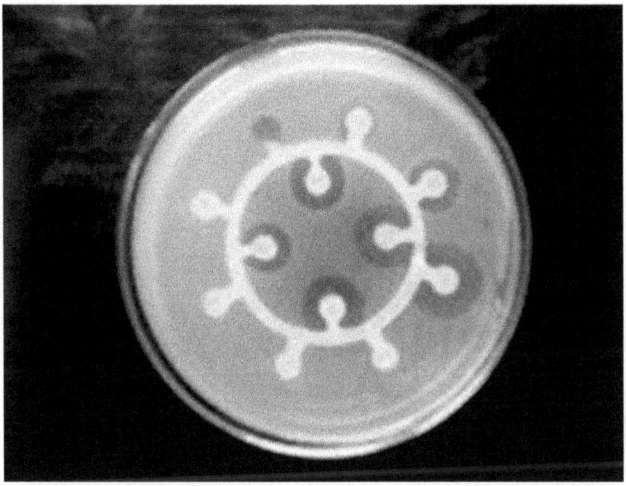

Figure 11.1: Disc Diffusion Method.

Result

The zones of inhibition can be graded as ++++, +++, ++, + or R (resistant) for no zones depending on the diameter of zone. Commercially available disc manufacturers provide the zone charts and these charts can be used for interpretation of results.

Part 2

Chapter 12

Introduction of Fungi

Introduction

The branch of botany that deals with the study of fungi is called mycology (Greek *mycos* = mushroom, *logos* = discourse). Alexopoulos and Mims in 1979, the fungi should be kept in a kingdom myceteae, separated from plant kingdom.

Outline about Fungi

- The fungi are eukaryotic, non-motile, non-photosynthetic organism.
- Out of 250,000 species only 150 species of fungi is pathogenic for animals and human.
- The optimum pH of fungi is 6 but can tolerate acidic pH. Fungi can grow well in 25°C temperature.
- In the laboratory media, growth of fungi is very slow. Example. Zygomycetes growth occur in media 2-3 days whereas dermatophytes takes more time around 3-5 weeks.
- Morphological fungal forms are moulds, yeasts and dimorphs. Moulds are filamentous with branching hyphae 2-10 µm in diameter whereas yeast are oval or spherical or elongated cells, 3to 5 µm in diameter and produces bacteria like colonies. Dimorphic fungi occur in both forms moulds and yeasts.
- They are yeast like in animal tissue at 37°C and moulds form in the natural environment at 25°C.
- Fungi grow on Sabouraud dextrose agar media.
- Dermatophytes are pathogens which cause ringworm in animals and humans.

Characteristics of Fungi

General characteristics of fungi are as follows:

- ✰ Fungi are eukaryotic organisms.
- ✰ They are non-vascular organisms.
- ✰ They reproduce by means of spores.
- ✰ They are typical non-motile.
- ✰ Depending on the species and conditions both sexual and asexual spores may be produced.
- ✰ Fungi exhibit the phenomena of alteration of generation.
- ✰ The vegetative body of the fungi may be unicellular or composed of microscopic threads called hyphae.
- ✰ The structure of cell wall is similar to plants but chemically the fungi cell wall is composed of chitin.
- ✰ Fungi are heterotrophic organisms.
- ✰ Fungi store their food as starch.
- ✰ Biosynthesis of chitin occurs in fungi.
- ✰ The nuclei of the fungi are very small.
- ✰ During mitosis the nuclear envelope is not dissolved.
- ✰ Nutrition in fungi – they are saprophytes, or parasites or symbionts.
- ✰ Reproduction in fungi is fungi are both by sexual and asexual means.

Classification of Fungi

Based on the spore case in which the spores are produced fungi are classified into four divisions.

Division Ascomycota: Sac Fungi

The sac-fungi produce spores in small cup-shaped sacs called asci, that's why the name ascomycota. The mature sac fungi spores are known as ascospores, Yeast is the most common one-celled fungi. Yeast reproduces through asexual process called budding. The buds form at the side of the parent cell. Example: *Aspergillus, Claviceps, Neurospora.*

Division Basidiomycota: Club Fungi

Basidiomycota includes the mushrooms; the spores are borne on a club-shaped spore case called basidium. Example: *Agaricus* (mushroom), *Ustilago* (smut), and *Puccinia* (rust fungus).

Division Zygomycota: Zygote forming Fungi

These fungi are usually found on cheese, bread, and other decaying food. They are zygote forming fungi, hence the name zygomycota. The spores are produced in round-shaped case called sporangium. Example: *Mucor, Rhizopus* and *Albugo.*

Division Deuteromycota: Imperfect Fungi

These organisms are known as imperfect fungi because they lack sexual reproduction. They reproduce by asexual spores known as conidia. Most of the fungi cause diseases to humans like ringworm. Economically important imperfect fungi are *Penicillium* and *Aspergillus*.

Habitate and Nutrition of Fungi

As known that fungi are found everywhere. They are unable to synthesize their food molecules due to lack of chlorophyll pigments. So they are either parasites or saprophytes. Most of the fungi are saprophytes only some of the fungi are symbiotic parasites. Parasitic fungi obtained their nutrition from host and die with the death of the host. They cannot be grown artificially on a synthetic medium. Such types of fungi are called *obligate parasites*. Some fungi, which are parasitic but after death of the host, are able to get the nutrition or food from the decaying body of the host are called *facultative saprophytes*. Those fungi, which always take their nutrition from the decaying organic material (such as food, gems, bread, fruits and decaying leather etc), are called obligate saprophytes and those fungi which are saprophytes but can live parasitically under some condition are called *facultative parasites*.

Parasites which grown on host cell surface and absorb their food via haustoria are known as *ectoparasites* and those which enter into the tissue of the host are called *endoparasites*.

Fungi that decompose or decay dead organic matters are important to all forms of life because they restock the environment with inorganic nutrient matter, essential for host (Plant and animal), otherwise the ecosystem will collapse.

Structure of Fungi

Structure of the fungi is simple, unicellular, uninucleated forms such as yeast and synchytrium, a thread like structure called mycelium (mycelia-plural), which made up of tubular filaments called hyphae (hypha-singular). The hypha is bound by a fungus cell wall chitin, chitin is a nitrogenous polysaccharides. By hyphae the fungus develops a large surface, from which it can secrete digestive enzymes on food products, which can be easily absorbed by fungi. The protoplasm of the hypha may be continuous without septa, is called aseptate hypha or is with septa (cross-wall) is called septate hypha. Aseptate hypha is multinucleated tube like structure called coenocytes. Example zygomycetes. In aseptate hyphae, septa are formed when reproductive structures are produced. In septate hypha, septa have central pore and called perforated or porus septa but in some times pore may be absent in the septa called nonporous septa.

Reproduction Process of Fungi

Fungi exhibit **two** major modes of reproduction - Asexual and sexual.

Fungal reproduction is complex process. Fungi reproduce sexually and/or asexually. Perfect fungi reproduce both sexually and asexually, while imperfect fungi reproduce only asexually (by mitosis).

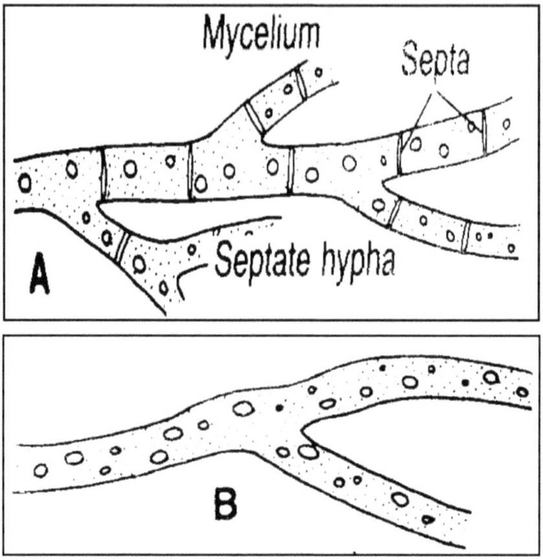

Figure 12.1: Structure of Fungi.
A: Septate hypha and B: Aseptate hypha.

In both sexual and asexual reproduction, fungi produce spores that disperse from the parent organism by either floating on the wind or hitching a ride on an animal. Fungal spores are smaller and lighter than plant seeds.

I) Asexual Reproduction

Fungi reproduce asexually by fragmentation, budding, or producing spores. Fragments of hyphae can grow new colonies. Mycelial fragmentation occurs when a fungal mycelium separates into pieces with each component growing into a separate mycelium.

In yeast form buds. During budding, a bulge forms on the side of the cell, the nucleus divides mitotically, and the bud ultimately detaches itself from the mother cell.

The most common mode of asexual reproduction is through the formation of asexual spores, which are produced by one parent only (through mitosis) and are genetically identical to that parent. Spores allow fungi to expand their distribution and colonize new environments. They may be released from the parent thallus, either outside or within a special reproductive sac called a sporangium.

There are many types of asexual spores.

Zoospores

They are uni-flagellated, motile spores produced inside structures called zoosporangia. These spores do not have a cell wall. Such spores are produced in lower fungi such as Achyla and Saprolegnia.

Sporagiospores

These are non-motile spores produced inside structures called sporangia in fungi such as Rhizopus and Mucor. These spores are dispersed by wind.

Chlamydospores

These are thick walled resting spores which arise directly from hyphal cells. They store reserve food.

Oidia

These are spore like structures formed by the breaking up of hypha cells. They do not store reserve food and hence cannot survive under unfavourable conditions. Such spores are produced in Rhizopus.

Conidia

These are non-motile spores produced singly or in chains at the tip of the hypha branches that are called conidiophores. Such spores are produced in fungi like Aspergillus and Penicillium.

II) Sexual Reproduction

Sexual reproduction is reduced in fungi and take palce by two fusing gametes.

It includes three stages.

A) Planogametic Copulation

In this process, fusion of two gametes of opposite sex or strains takes place. One or both of the fusing gamete are motile. It results in the formation of a diploid zygote. This process is usually of two types.

I) Isogamy

Fusing gametes are morphologically similar but physiologically dissimilar called isogamy.

II) Heterogamy

Fusing gametes are morphologically and physiologically different, the process is called heterogamy. Heterogamous reproduction is two types.

a) Anisogamy

Fusion of two gametes, male gametes are smaller and active compare to female gametes (Larger and less active). *e.g. Allomyces.*

b) Oogamy

The gametes are produced inside the morphologically different gametangia.

The male gametangia are smaller and called antheridium, while female gametangia are larger and called oogonium. The antheridium bears smaller, active and motile gametes known as sperm while oogonium is non-motile, large egg.

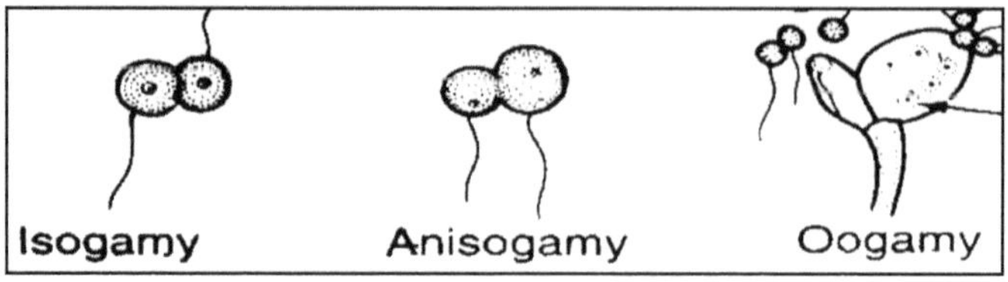

Planogametic copulation

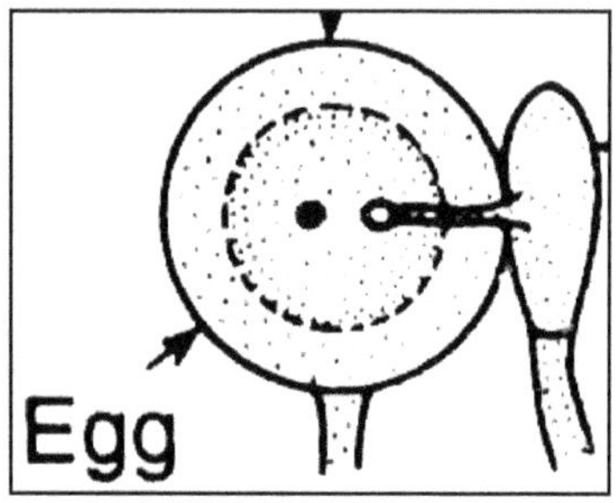

Gametangial contact

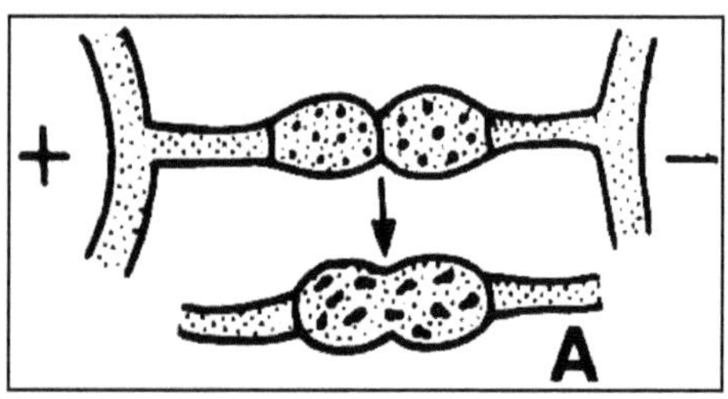

Gametangial copulation

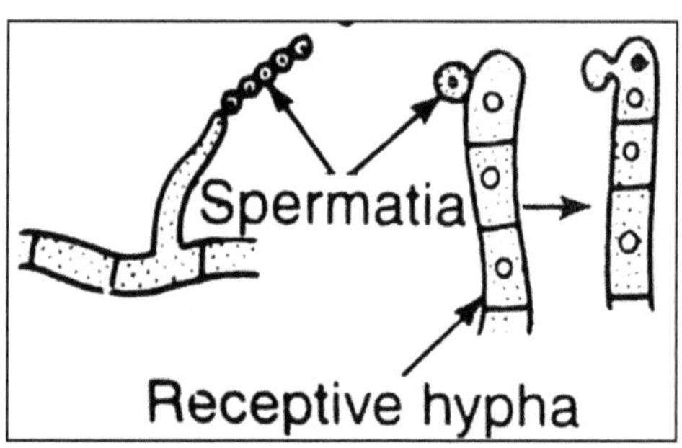

Spermatization

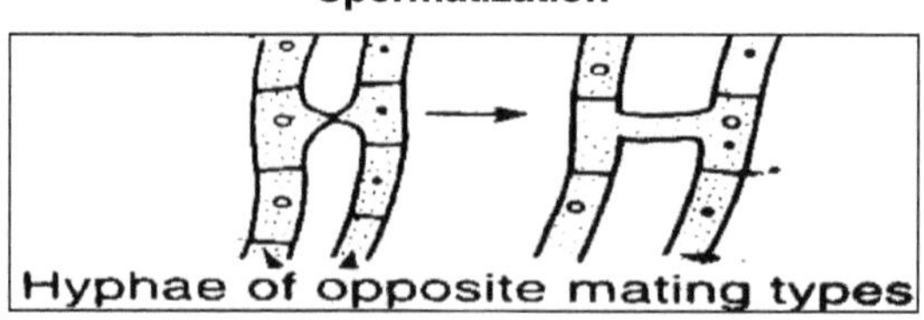

Somatogamy

Figure 12.2: Showing different Method of Sexual Reproduction.

B) Gametengial Contact

In this process, gamete bearing structure called gametangia come closer to each other and develop a fertilization tube through which the male gametes migrates into the female gametangium, *e.g. Albugo.*

C) Gametengial Copulation

In this process, the gametangia fuse with each other, lose their identity and develop into a zygospore, *e.g. Mucor, Rhizopus.*

D) Spermatisation

In some fungi such as Puccinia tiny unicellular spore like structure called spermatia are formed. They get transferred to female gametangia through various ways.

E) Somatogamy

This takes place in fungi where gametes are not formed. In such fungi anastamoses takes place between somatic structures bearing nuclei of different percentage, whereby nuclei of one passess into corresponding somatic cell by dissolving the wall, thus establishing a dikaryotic condition. *e.g. Agaricus.*

Part 3

Chapter 13

Introduction to Virus

Viral nucleic acid contains around 4 to 400 genes. The nucleic acid is either DNA or RNA, each nucleic acid have unique features such as.

Deoxyribonucleic Acid (DNA)

- ☆ Nucleic acid either single stranded and/or double stranded.
- ☆ Circular or linear.
- ☆ Glycosylated and/or methylated.
- ☆ Purine and/or pyrimidine base present.

Ribonucleic Acid (RNA)

- ☆ Single stranded and/or double stranded.
- ☆ Segmented or Non-segmented.
- ☆ Purine and/or pyrimidine base present.
- ☆ Folding pattern.

Capsid

- ☆ It is the protein coat of the virus.
- ☆ It is a complex and highly organized.
- ☆ Subunits called protomeres aggregate to form capsomeres which in turn aggregate to form the capsid.

Envelope

Envelope is composed of lipid, protein and carbohydrate. Which lies to the outside of the capsid and contains a mosaic of antigens from the host and the virus.

Spikes

- ✰ These are glycoprotein projections.
- ✰ Spikes/projection have enzymatic and/or adsorption and/or hemagglutinating activity.
- ✰ They arise from the envelope and are highly antigenic.

Morphological Structure of Animal Viruses

Virus Symmetry

1. Icosahedral

Isometric symmetry of the viruses, the capsid consists of 20 is dentical triangular faces, which are joined along the edges. In such formation, the capsid acquires 12 vertices (corners) and 30 edges.Capsomeres are the morphological unit of capsid and their number varies and the formula for calculation of the numbers are

$N = 10(n-1)^2 + 2$ **or** $N = 10T + 2$

whereas,

N = Number of capsomers on one edge of triangular face

T = Triangulation numbers

e.g. If $n = 6$	$T = 25$
$N = 10(n-1)^2 + 2$	$N = 10T + 2$
$N = 10(6-1)^2 + 2$	$N = 10 \times 25 + 2$
$N = 252$	$N = 252$

2. Helical

The protomeres are not grouped in capsomeres, but are bound to each other so as to form a ribbon-like structure. This structure folds into a helix because the protomeres are thicker at one end than at the other. The diameter of the helical capsid is determined by characteristics of its protomeres, while its length is determined by the length of the nucleic acid it encloses.*e.g. Paramyxoviridae, orthomyxoviridae, coronaviridae.*

3. Complex

Symmetry *poxviruses* and *rhabdoviruses* do not fit into either of two a foresaid types. In this respect, their symmetry is complex.

Chemical Structure

The essential components of infectious virus particles are Nucleic acid and protein.

Nucleic Acid

Virus contains only one type of nucleic acid, either single or double stranded DNA or RNA. In DNA viruses the genome consists of single molecules whereas

RNA virus consist segmented genome and consist of several molecules. Single molecules of nucleic acid are called *monopartile* and viral genes contain multiple molecules of nucleic acid called *multipartile.*

All viral genome are haploid (contain one copy of each gene) except *Retrovirus* genome (Diploid). DNA viruses' genomes are linear or circular configuration but in RNA viruses are linear genome.

All DNA virus genome is double stranded except Parvovirus and *Circovirus. Hepadavirus* has partially double stranded genome.

All RNA viruses have single stranded genome except *Rreovirus* and *Bbirnavirus.* The size of DNA of different viruses ranges from 1.7kb (*Circovirus*) to 200 kb (*Poxvirus*).

The size of RNA of single stranded viruses varies from 1.7 to 21 kb while in case of ds size varies from 18 to 27 kb.

Molecular weight of DNA of different viruses varies from $1\text{-}200\times10^6$.

Molecular weight of RNA of different viruses varies from $2\text{-}15\times10^6$.

RNA viruses are positive or negative sense. The positive sense RNA viruses are infectious because viral RNA itself act as a m-RNA.

Negative sense RNA is not infectious because RNA cannot function as m-RNA and required to produce positive sense RNA with a virion associated transcriptase. Retrovirus is positive sense RNA virus but is not infectious because replication of RNA occurs only after production of proviral DNA by virus associated reverse transcriptase. Number of segment of RNA viruses may vary from 2 to 12.

Protein

Proteins form a major part of most of the viruses and around 40-65 per cent constituent of the viruses is protein. Viruses contain several types of proteins like as FMD virus contains four types of proteins VP_1, VP_2, VP_3 and VP_4.

Virus coated protein are called structural protein and they form the part of the viruses and many viruses induced non-structural proteins are found in cells infected with the viruses.

Number of the structural protein is also varying with the types of viruses.

Some enveloped viruses (*Orthmyxovirus/Paramyxovirus/Rhabdoviruses*) the inner surface of the lipid layer and contains large numbers of glycosylated protein called matrix protein. The peplomer of the enveloped viruses contains glycoproteins which act as antigenic determinants.

Function of Structural Protein

To protect the viral nucleic acid. The structural proteins are antigenic in nature and responsible for production of protective antibody. Non- structural proteins of the viruses are mostly the early proteins and are required for virus multiplication.

Enzyme

Viruses do not have any metabolic enzymes, which is essential for replication. Some virus contain enzymes, reverse transcriptase enzymes of Retroviruses, Poxvirus carry a number of unique enzymes for processing RNA transcripts and replication of their genome. These viral enzymes are mostly the structural proteins, but some viral enzymes can synthesized as early protein.

Lipid and Carbohydrate

The envelope of viruses possess lipid and carbohydrate are mostly derived from host cells. Carbohydrate is also the major part of the peplomers. Lipid constitutes 25–35 per cent of the dry weight of most of the enveloped viruses. The lipid in the viral envelope is phospholipid.

Chapter 14

Classification of Viruses

The History of Virus Taxonomy

The object of virus classification is to make a systematic ordered arrangement of the viruses that have similarities and differences. The first discoveries of viruses were made on the basis of their size (small) as assessed by filterability and no other measurement made at that time. Most of the studies were centred on their ability to cause infections and diseases. Such system have dificiencies *e.g.* The same virus produces different disease syndromes in different hosts, different strains of the same virus can produce different syndromes in the same host and different viruses can produces the same pictures. Epidemeological data based classification was also tried earlier.

The most important criteria for classification are

I) Virion structure

II) Genome of the viruses

III) Mode of replication

Bawden in 1941-50, proposed first time that viruses grouped on the basis of shared virion properties.

The International Committee on Taxonomy of Viruses (ICTV)

Against this background, in 1966 the the International Committee on Nomenclature of Viruses (ICNV) was established at the International Congress of Microbiology in Moscow. At that time, Virologists already sensed a need for a single, universal taxonomic scheme. There was dispute that the viruses were isolated from humans, animals, plants and invertebrates should be classified in a single system and that this system should separate the viruses from all other biological entities. The International Committee on Nomenclature of Viruses (ICNV) become the

International Committee on Taxonomy of Viruses (ICTV) in 1973. Today ICTV operates under the auspices of the Virology division of the international union of Microbiological Societies. In the ICTV have six sub-committees, 45 study groups and more than 400 virologists.

ICTV develop universal scheme, Virion characteristics are considered and weight by these criteria to division into the families, in some cases sub-families and genera. Now three orders (Mononegavirales, Nidovirales, and Caudovirales) have been approved. More than 1550 viruses species belonging to 3 orders, 56 families, 9 sub-families and 233 genera are recognised

Classification

Viruses are classed into 7 types of genes and each of which has its own families of viruses, which in turn have differing replication strategies themselves. David Baltimore, a Nobel Prize-winning biologist, devised a system called the Baltimore Classification System to classify different viruses based on their unique replication strategy. There are seven different replication strategies based on this system (Baltimore Class I, II, III, IV, V, VI, and VII).

Class 1: Double-Stranded DNA Viruses

This type of virus usually must enter the host nucleus before it is able to replicate. Some of these viruses require host cell polymerases to replicate their genome, while others, such as adenoviruses or herpes viruses, encode their own replication factors. However, in either cases, replication of the viral genome is highly dependent on a cellular state permissive to DNA replication and, thus, on the cell cycle. The virus may induce the cell to forcefully undergo cell division, which may lead to transformation of the cell and, ultimately, cancer. An example of a family within this classification is the *Adenoviridae.*

There is only one well-studied example in which a class 1 family of viruses does not replicate within the nucleus. This is the *Poxvirus* family, which comprises highly pathogenic viruses that infect vertebrates.

Class 2: Single-Stranded DNA Viruses

Viruses that fall under this category include ones that are not as well-studied, but still do pertain highly to vertebrates. Two examples include the *Circoviridae* and *Parvoviridae*. They replicate within the nucleus, and form a double-stranded DNA intermediate during replication. A human *Circovirus* called TTV is included within this classification and is found in almost all humans, infecting them asymptomatically in nearly every major organ.

Class 3: Double-Stranded RNA Viruses

Like most viruses with RNA genomes, double-stranded RNA viruses do not rely on host polymerases for replication to the extent that viruses with DNA genomes do. Double-stranded RNA viruses are not as well-studied as other classes. This class includes two major families, the *Reoviridae* and *Birnaviridae*. Replication is monocistronic and includes individual, segmented genomes, meaning that each of the genes codes for only one protein, unlike other viruses, which exhibit more complex translation.

Classes 4 and 5: Single-Stranded RNA Viruses

These viruses consist of two types, however both share the fact that replication is primarily in the cytoplasm, and that replication is not as dependent on the cell cycle as that of DNA viruses. This class of viruses is also one of the most-studied types of viruses, alongside the double-stranded DNA viruses.

Class 4: Single-Stranded RNA Viruses - Positive-Sense

The positive-sense RNA viruses and indeed all genes defined as positive-sense can be directly accessed by host ribosomes to immediately form proteins. These can be divided into two groups, both of which replicate in the cytoplasm:

- ✰ Viruses with polycistronic mRNA where the genome RNA forms the mRNA and is translated into a polyprotein product that is subsequently cleaved to form the mature proteins. This means that the gene can utilize a few methods in which to produce proteins from the same strand of RNA, all in the sake of reducing the size of its gene.
- ✰ Viruses with complex transcription, for which subgenomic mRNAs, ribosomal frameshifting and proteolytic processing of polyproteins may be used. All of which are different mechanisms with which to produce proteins from the same strand of RNA.

Examples of this class include the families *Coronaviridae, Flaviviridae* and *Picornaviridae.*

Class 5: Single-Stranded RNA Viruses – (Negative-sense)

The negative-sense RNA viruses and indeed all genes defined as negative-sense cannot be directly accessed by host ribosomes to immediately form proteins.

Instead, they must be transcribed by viral polymerases into the "readable" complementary positive-sense. These can also be divided into two groups:

- ✰ Viruses containing non-segmented genomes for which the first step in replication is transcription from the negative-stranded genome by the viral RNA-dependent RNA polymerase to yield monocistronic mRNAs that code for the various viral proteins. A positive-sense genome copy that serves as template for production of the negative-strand genome is then produced. Replication is within the cytoplasm.
- ✰ Viruses with segmented genomes for which replication occurs in the cytoplasm and for which the viral RNA-dependent RNA polymerase produces monocistronic mRNAs from each genome segment.

Examples: *Orthomyxoviridae, Paramyxoviridae, Bunyaviridae, Filoviridae* and *Rhabdoviridae*

Class 6: Positive-Sense Single-Stranded RNA Viruses that Replicate through a DNA Intermediate

A well-studied family of this class of viruses include the retroviruses. One defining feature is the use of reverse transcriptase to convert the positive-sense RNA into DNA. Instead of using the RNA for templates of proteins, they use DNA to create the templates, which is spliced into the host genome using integrase. Replication can then commence with the help of the host cell's polymerases

Class 7: Double-stranded DNA Viruses that Replicate through a Single-Stranded RNA Intermediate

This small group of viruses, exemplified by the Hepatitis B virus, have a double-stranded, gapped genome that is subsequently filled in to form a covalently closed circle (ccc DNA) that serves as a template for production of viral mRNAs and a subgenomic RNA. The pregenome RNA serves as template for the viral reverse transcriptase and for production of the DNA genome.

Toxonomy System

DNA Viruses

Double Stranded DNA Viruses

Family	*Sub-family*	*Genus*	*Species*
Poxviridae	Chondropoxvirinae	Orthopoxvirus	Vaccinia virus
		Capripoxvirus	Sheeppox virus
		Leporipoxvirus	Myxoma virus
		Suispoxvirus	Swinepox virus
		Molluscipoxvirus	Molluscum contagiosum virus
		Avipoxvirus	Fowlpox virus
		Yatapoxvirus	Yabamonkey tumor virus
		Parapoxvirus	Orf virus
	Entamopoxvirinae	Entamopoxvirus genera A,B,C	Insect virus
Asfarviridae		Asfivirus	African swine fever virus
Iridoviridae		Ranavirus	Frog virus 3 } No veterinary importance
		Lymphosystivirus	Flounder virus } No veterinary importance
Herpesviridae	Alphherpesvirinae	Simplexvirus	Human herpesvirus 1
		Varicellovirus	Human herpesvirus 3
		Marke's disease virus	Marke's disease virus
		Infectious larynotracheitis virus	Gallid herpesvirus 1

Family	Sub-family	Genus	Species
	Betaherpesvirinae	Cytomegalovius	Human herpesvirus 5
		Muromegalovirus	Mouse herpesvirus 2 Cavid herpesvirus 2
		Roseolovirus	Human herpesvirus 6
	Gammaherpesvirinae	Lymphocryptovirus	Human herpesvirus 4
		Rhadinovirus	Allelophine herpesvirus 1
Adeniviridae		Mastadenovirus	Human adenovirus 2
		Aviadenovirus	Fowl adenovirus 1
		Atadenovirus	Ovine adenovirus 287
Papovaviridae		Polyomavirus	Murine polyomavirus
		Papillomavirus	Rabbit papilloma virus

Single Stranded DNA Viruses

Family	Sub-family	Genus	Species
Parvoviridae	Parvovirinae	Parvovirus	Minute virus of mice
		Erythrovirus	B-19virus
		Dependovirus	Adeno associated virus 2
Circoviridae		Circovirus	Cheken anemia virus

DNA Dependent RNA Reverse Transcribing Viruses

Family	Sub-family	Genus	Species
Hepadnaviridae	Parvovirinae	Arthohepdna virus	Hepatitis B virus
		Avihepadna virus	Duck hepatitis B virus
Retroviridae		Alpharetrovirus	Avian leukosis virus
		Betaretrovirus	Mouse mammary tumor virus
		Gammaretrovirus	Murine leukemiavirus
		Delata retrovirus	Bovine leukemi virus
		Lenti virus	Human immunodeficiency virus

RNA Viruses

Double Stranded RNA Virus

Family	Sub-family	Genus	Species
Reoviridae		Orthoreovirus	Reo virus 3
		Orbivirus	Blue tongue virus 1
		Rotavirus	Simian rotavirus SA11
Birnaviridae		Avibirnavirus	Infectious bural disease virus
		Aquabirnavirus	Infectious pancreatic necrosis virus of fish

Single Stranded DNA Viruses

Family	Sub-family	Genus	Species
Parvoviridae	Parvovirinae	Parvovirus	Minute virus of mice
		Erythrovirus	B19 VIRUS
		Dependovirus	Adeno associated virus 2
Circoviridae		Circovirus	Chicken anemia virus

Single Stranded Negative Sense RNA Viruses

Family	Sub-family	Genus	Species
Order-Mononegavirales	Paramyxovirinae	Respirovirus	Human parainfluenza virus 1
Paramyxoviridae		Morbillivirus	Measles virus
		Rubella virus	Mumps virus
	Pneumovirinae	Pneumovirus	Human respiratory syncytial virus
		Metapneumovirus	Turkey rhinotracheitis virus
Order-Mononegavirales		Vesiculovirus	Vesicular stomatitis virus
Rhabdoviridae		Lyssavirus	Rabies virus
		Ephimerovirus	Bovine ephemeral fever virus
Order-Mononegavirales		Marburh like virus	Marburh like virus
Filoviridael		Ebola like virus	Ebola virus
Order-Mononegavirales Bornavirus		Bornavirus	Borna disease virus
Orthomyxoviridae		Influenza virus A	Influenza virus A
		Influenza virus B	Influenza virus B
		Influenza virus C	Influenza virus C
		Thogotovirus	Thogotovirus
Bunyaviridae		Bunyavirus	Bunyamwera virus
		Hantnavirus	Hantaana virus
		Nairovirus	Naiirobi sheep disease virus
		Phlebovirus	Sandy fever Sicilian virus
Arenaviridae		Arenavirus	Lymphocytic choriomeningitis virus

Single Stranded Positive Sense RNA Viruses

Family	*Sub-family*	*Genus*	*Species*
Order-Nidovirales		Coronavirus	Avian infectious bronchitis virus
Coronaviridae		Torovirus	Berbe virus
Order-Nidovirales Arteriviridae		Arterivirus	Equine arteritis virus
Picornaviridae		Enterovirus	Poliovirus
		RRhinovirus	Human rhinovirus 1A
		Hepatovirus	Hepatitis A virus
		Cardovirus	Encephalomyocarditis virus
		Aphthovirus	Foot and mouth disease virus O
Caliciviridae		Vesivirus	Vesicular exanthema of swine virus
		Lagovirus	Rabbit hemorrhagic disease virus
Astroviridae		Astrovirus	Human astrovirus 1
Togoviridae		Alphavirus	Sindbis virus
		Rubivirus	Rubella virus
Flaviviridae		Flavivirus	Yellow fever virus
		Pestivirus	Bovine viral diarrhea virus
		Hepacivirus	Hepatitis C virus
Subviral agents: Prions			Scrapie prion
Satellites		Deltavirus	Hepatitis delta virus

Different Group of Viruses

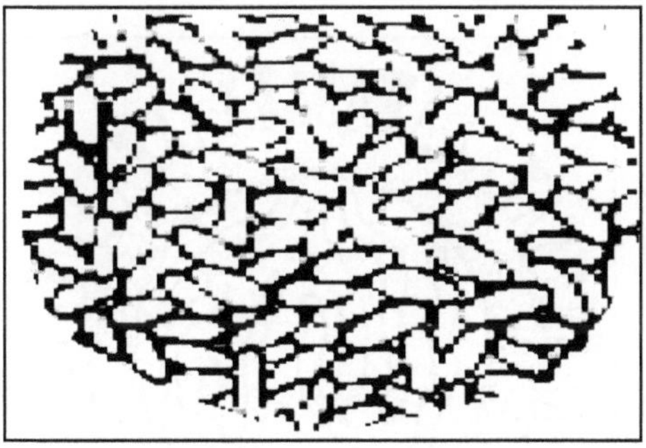

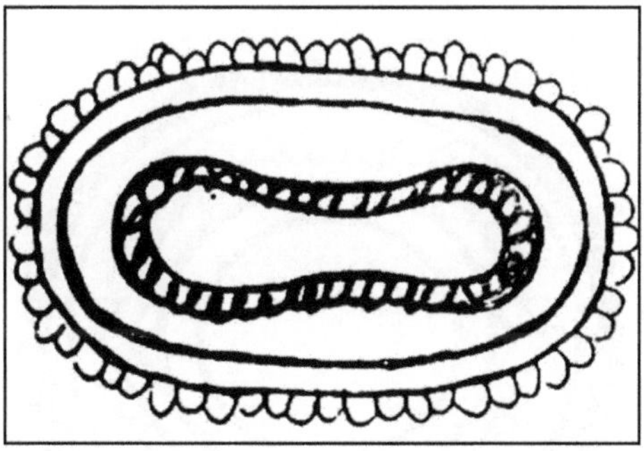

Poxvirus

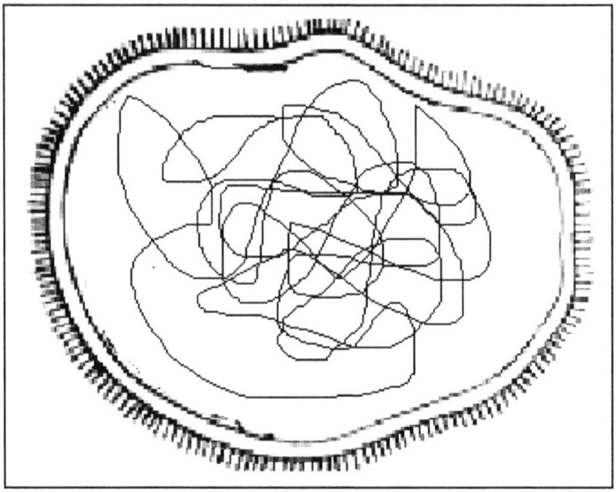

Paramyxovirus

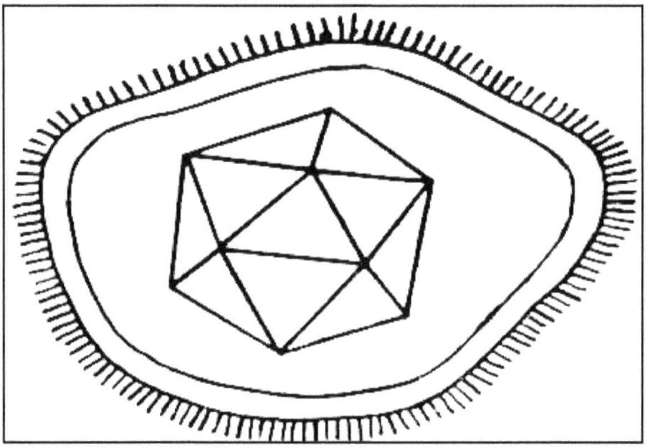

Herpesvirus

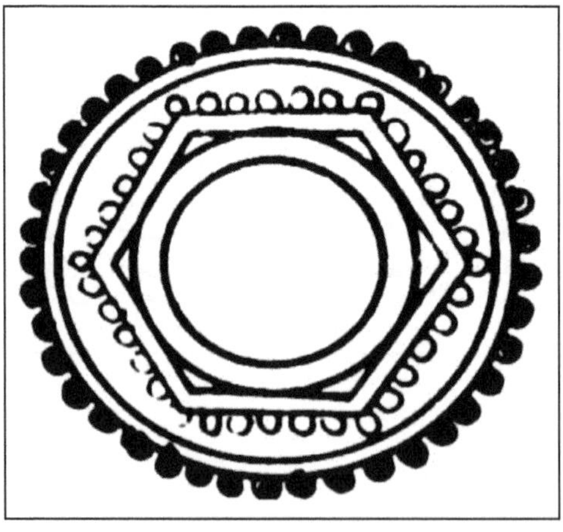

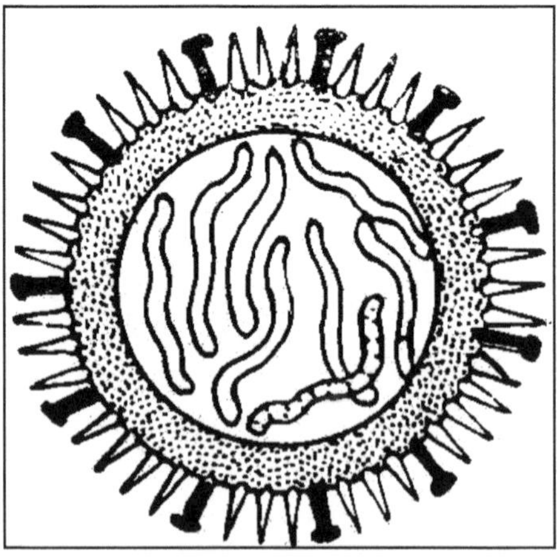

Retrovirus ***Orthomyxovirus***

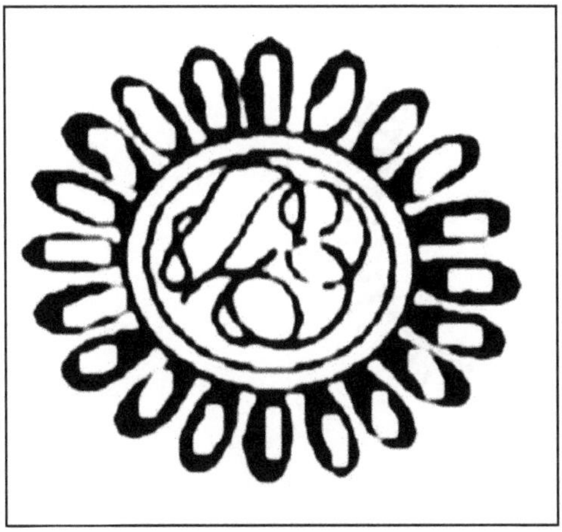

Coronavirus

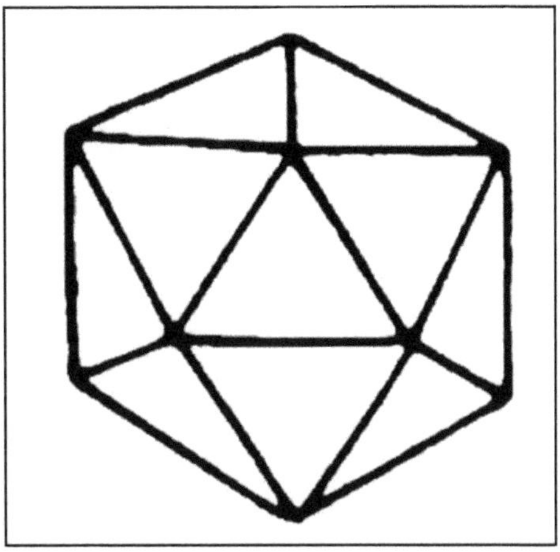

Adenovirus

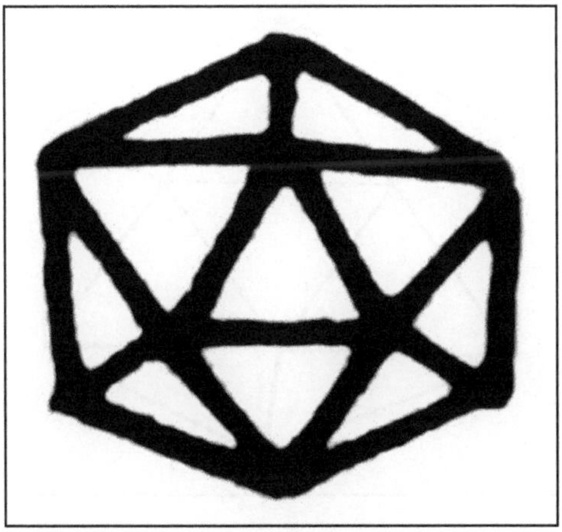

Picornavirus

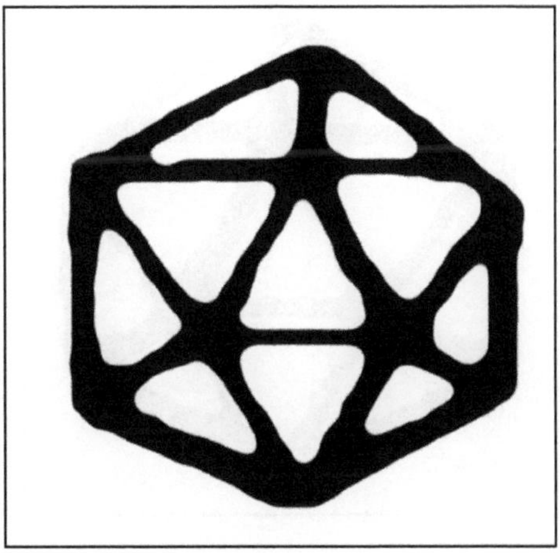

Parvovirus

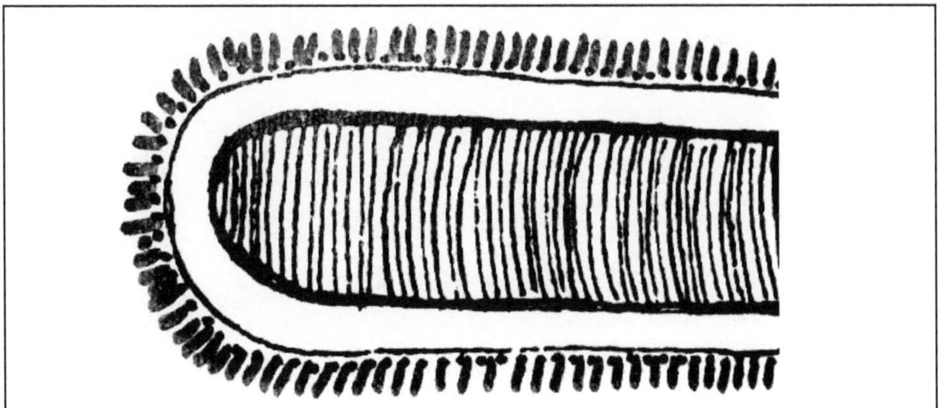

Rhabdovirus

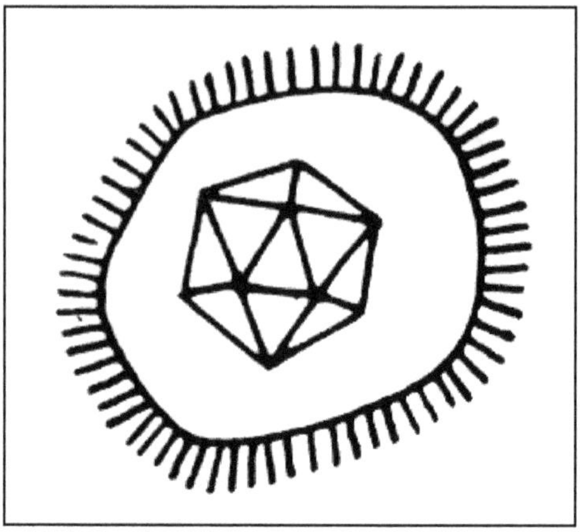

Togavirus

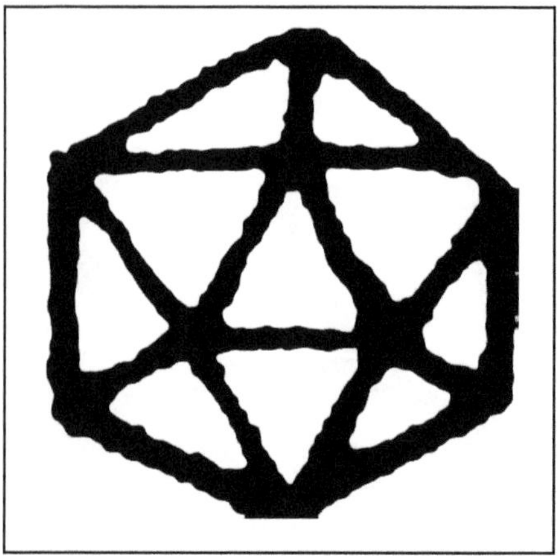

Asfarviridae

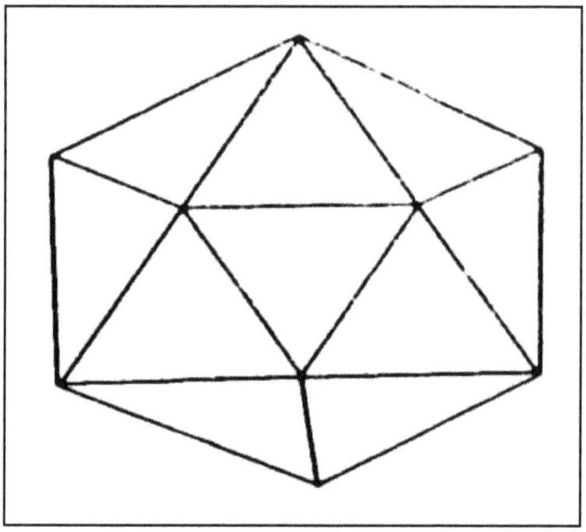

Papillomaviridae

Chapter 15

Viral Replication

Viral replication process occurs in following steps.

1) Adsorption
2) Penetration
3) Uncoating
4) Transcription
5) Translation
   - ☆ Replication of viral nucleic acid
6) Maturation
7) Release of virus

1) Adsorption

Viruses can enter cells via phagocytosis, viropexis or adsorption. Adsorption is the most common process and the most highly specific process. It occurs by interaction of virus surface protein with a highly specific receptor site on the surface of the cell.

2) Penetration

This occurs by one or more processes.

- ☆ **Enveloped viruses** fuse their envelope with the membrane of the host cell. This involves local digestion of the viral and cellular membranes, fusion of the membranes and concomitant release of the nucleocapsid into the cytoplasm.
- ☆ **Non- Enveloped or Naked viruses** bind to receptor sites on the cellular membrane, digest the membrane and enter into the cytoplasm intact.

☆ **Both Non- Enveloped and enveloped viruses** can be ingested by phagocytic cells. However, in this process they enter the cytoplasm enclosed in a cytoplasmic membrane derived from the phagocytic cell.

3) Uncoating

After penetration process,uncoating occurs by digest the capsid with the cellular proteolytic enzymes. Uncoating process always occurs in the cytoplasm of the host cell.

The period of the replication cycle between the end of the uncoating stage and maturation of new viral particles is termed the ***eclipse period***. Thus during the eclipse stage, no complete viral particles can be viewed within the cell.

4) Transcription

All DNA viruses transcription are occurs in nucleaous of host cells except poxvirus and cellular DNA dependent RAN polymerase performs the transcription process, whereas poxvirus transcription occur in the cytoplasm and virion associated DNA dependent RNA polymerase is involve in transcription.

Parvovirus (ss DNA virus) a complementary strands to form ds DNA with the help of cellular transcriptase.

All RNA viruses replication is occur in the host cell cytoplasm except *orthomyxoviruses* and retroviruses. RNA virus replication is more complicated than the DNA viruses.

In case of ss (+)RNA viruses directly transcribed to m-RNA, whereas ss (-)RNA viruses transcribed in to full length positive sense RNA strand by virion associated transcriptase.

In ss RNA with segmented genomes, each segment is transcribed to produce m-RNA.

The retroviruses, positive ssense ss RNA is not directly transcribed, there is reverse transcription of their nucleic acid in to ds DNA by the virion associated reverse transcriptase. The DNA is then integrated into the cellular DNA. The integrated viral DNA transcription of RNA occurs by the cellular transcriptase.

Reoviruses and *birnaviruses* (ds RNA virus) have segmented genome occur in the cytoplasm by a virion association RNA dependent RNA polymerease and each segment transcribed separately and one strand of each segment is used as a template for m-RNA.

5) Translation

In translation, viral m-RNA bind to ribosome and translated into protein. Translation occur in same ways as eukaryotic cell m-RNAs. Each m-RNA molecules bind to 40 s-ribosomal subunit at 5^I terminal end. The 60 s- ribosomal subunit bind together with methionyl t-RNA nad various initiation factors after that translation starts. The proteins translated from the early m-RNA of DNA viruses includes enzymes and proteins, which is required for viral nucleic acid replication and also required for suppression of host cell RNA and protein synthesis. The viral protein translated from the late m-RNA and Viral structural proteins.

In RNA viruses, non-structural proteins are formed by early m-RNAs whereas structural proteins are formed by late m-RNAs. RNA viruses (*Picornaviruses and Flaviviruses*) gemone act as single polycistronic m-RNA and translated into single poly protein, which is cleaved into smaller proteins by virion coded protease. The newly synthesized by virion proteins migrate to various sites (nucleous or cytoplasm) depending upon the viruses. The mechanism how to control the migration is not, exactly clear but suggested that it is depends on the structural features protein. For examples, in case of glycoproteins the polypeptides is translated on rough endoplasmic reticulum. Various post translational modification occur as the proteins move to Golgi complex and then to plasma-membrane.

Replication of Viral Nucleic Acid

Replication of viral nucleic acid is a complex process. The specific process depends on the nucleic acid types.

DNA replication depends upon the different viruses.

A. **Adenoviruses** – *Adenoviruses* DNA virus (linear ds DNA) required specialized terminal structure, cellular DNA polymerase and early *adenovirus* protein. Replication started from the end of double strand. Synthesis from 5^I to 3^I proceeds continually with displacement of original strand. The displaced strands serve as template in the formation of ds molecules by sysnthesis of complimentary DNA strand.

B. **Herpesviruses** - *Herpesviruses* replicate in the nucleus requires a large number of enzymes in DNA synthesis and rolling circle mechanisms involves in the later stages of the DNA replication.

C. **Papovaviruses** - The DNA of *papovaviruses* are circular and the replication is bidirectional and symmetrical, via cyclic intermediates.

D. **Parvoviruses** - *Parvovirus,* ss linear DNA viruses are replicated by cellular polymerases. First viral ss DNA is converted into ds DNA (replicative form). The ss DNA replication subsequently copying of the template strand of the replicative form.

E. **Poxviruses** – Replication occur in the cytoplasm depending on the virus coded proteins. Replication started at each end of the genome and involves a strand displacement mechanism with the formation of small DNA fragments.

F. **Hepadnaviruses** - Replication occur in the nucleus. The virion associated DNA polymerase converts the viral nucleic acid to a complete circular double strand DNA. Negative sense strand of the molecules is translated into a full- length pregenome RNA by the cellular RNA polymerase, which is encapsidated in viral cores together with the viral DNA polymerase. The DNA polymerase also have reverse transcriptase activity. By reverse transcription of the pregenome RNA, the negative sense strand is synthesized. A small RNA fragments from the 5I end of the pregenome

RNA is used to prime the synthesis of the positive sense DNA strand. For maturation of the virus, complete synthesis of the positive sense DNA strand is not necessary because *Hepadnavirus* genome contains ds DNA with a portion of single stranded DNA.

The genome of RNA viruses either ss or ds, +ve or –ve sense must carry the information for synthesis of polymerase. The RNA dependent RNA polymerase is necessary for replication of RNA viruses, which is not found in mammalian cells. All –ve sense RNA viruses contain virion polymerase, which iniciate synthesis of complementary RNA strand of +ve sense. In case of +ve sense virion RNA the complementary RNA is of –ve sense from a single complementary RNA template several RNA molecules can be transcribed and each RNA transcript is the product of a separate bound polymerase molecules. The replication intermediate, which consist of several +ve sense ssRNA strands by separate molecules of RNA dependent RNA polymerase. Initiation of replication of some of the RNA viruses like *calcivirus, picornavirus etc.* required a VPg protein as primer and is covalently bound to the 5^{I} terminus of the +ve and –ve RNA strands, but not to m-RNA.

The ds RNA viruses (***reovirus***) replication, genome is conservative because the parental ds RNA remains sequestered in a sub – viral particles. The +ve sense RNA strand synthesized by a virion associated ds RNA dependent RNA polymerase and is then function as m-RNA or template RNA for synthesis of ds RNA progeny.

The ***retroviruses*** although +ve sense RNA but there is reverse transcription occurs via involvement of DNA intermediate, not like the other +ve sense RNA viruses. The virion associated RNA dependent RNA polymerese (reverse transcriptase) makes ss DNA copy by using t-RNA molecules as a primer. The reverse transcriptase removes the parental RNA molecules from the DNA-RNA hybrid. The –ve sense ss DNA intermediate is converted into linear ds DNA, which contains an additional sequence known as the long terminal repeat (LTR) at each end. The double stranded DNA is then migrated to the nucleus and integrated into cellular DNA in the form of proviral DNA.

6/7) Maturation and Release

☆ **Non-enveloped or Naked viruses** -Maturation consists of two main processes: there is assembly of the capsid, and its association with the nucleic acid. Maturation of the virion occurs at the site of nucleic acid replication. After they are assembled into mature viruses, naked virions may become concentrated in large numbers at the site of maturation, forming inclusion bodies. Naked virions are released in different ways, which depend on the virus and the cell type. Generally, RNA-containing naked viruses are released rapidly after maturation and there is little intracellular accumulation; therefore, these viruses do not form predominant inclusion bodies. On the other hand, DNA-containing naked icosahedral viruses that mature in the nucleus do not reach the cell surface as rapidly, and are released when the cells undergo autolysis or in some cases are extruded without lysis. In either case they tend to accumulate within the infected cells over a long period of time. Thus, they generally produce highly visible inclusion bodies.

- ☆ **Enveloped viruses** -In the maturation of enveloped viruses, a capsid must first be assembled around the nucleic acid to form the nucleocapsid, which is then surrounded by the envelope. During the assembly of the nucleocapsid, virus-coded envelope proteins are also synthesized. These migrate to the plasma membrane (if assembly occurs in the cytoplasm) or to the nuclear membrane (if assembly occurs in the nucleus) and become incorporated into that membrane. Envelopes are formed around the nucleocapsids by budding of cellular membranes.

  NOTE: Enveloped viruses will have an antigenic mosaicism characteristic of the virus and the host cell. Viruses are slowly and continuously released by the budding process with the results that: (a) the cell is not lysed; and (b) little intracellular accumulation of virus occurs; and (c) inclusion bodies are not as evident as with naked viruses.

- ☆ **Complex viruses** – *e.g. Poxvirus,* during maturation process forming multilayered membranes around the DNA. These layers differentiate into two membranes: The inner one contains the characteristic nucleoid, while the external one acquires the characteristic pattern of the surface of the virion. These form very characteristic cytoplasmic inclusion bodies. The viruses are generally released from the cell via cell lysis.

Chapter 16

Purification and Cultivation of Virus

Purification of Virus

There are different methods for purification of viruses.

- ☆ Viruses can be isolated from different centrifugation rate, at low speed centrifugation to eliminate the cell debris and supernatant is then centrifuge at high speed centrifugation.
- ☆ Purification of viruses with ammonium sulfate or polyethylene glycol.
- ☆ By using different concentration of sucrose gradients can be prepared. Easily and good separations of viruses and other particles of various sizes and densities.

Cultivation of Virus

As viruses are obligate intracellular parasites. They cannot be grown on any non-living or inanimate culture medium. There are following methods for virus cultivation.

1) Egg inoculation methods:
   - I. Allantoic sac inoculation
   - II. Amniotic sac inoculation
   - III. Yolk sac inoculation
   - IV. Chorioallantoic membrane (CAM) inoculation
   - V. Intraembryonic inoculation
   - VI. Intracerebral inoculation
   - VII. Intravenous inoculation

2) Animal inoculation
3) Tissue culture or cell culture
4) Cell-line

1) Egg Inoculation Methods

Embryonated chicken egg inoculations were fist used withpropagation of virus by Roux and Marfey in 1911. In 1931 Woodruff and Goodpasture cultivated fowl poxvirus on the chorioallantoic membrane. Burnet used chicken embryo for cultivation of viruses very extensively. Since that time and until mid 1950 almost all research and testing with viruses depended on animal or embryonated eggs for source of living tissue.

The methods of inoculation are as follows:

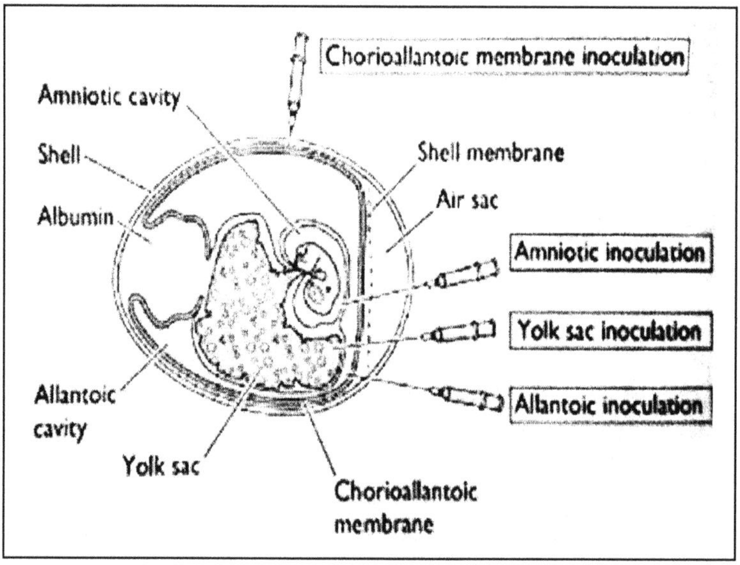

Figure 16.1: Embryonated Chicken Egg and different Routes of Virus Inoculation.

Allantoic Sac Inoculation

Procedure

- ☆ Candle the egg and mark the boundary of air sec with pencil.
- ☆ Select an area of the chorioallantoic membrane free of large blood vessels about 3mm below the base of the air sac.
- ☆ In this area make a pencil mark at the point for inoculation and other mark on air sac.
- ☆ Apply tincture of iodine at the site selected for making holes.

- ☆ Rubber cork with a pin dipped in tincture iodine is used for making holes on the air sac as well as on other selected site.
- ☆ Using a 1 ml tuberculin syringe fitted with a needle through a hole in the side of egg to a depth of about ¼ inch and deposite the inoculums.
- ☆ Withdraw the needle and seal the hole in the eggs with molten wax.

Amniotic Sac Inoculation

Procedure

- ☆ Candle 12-13 days old egg and make a pencil mark on the shell below the base of the air sac to lacate the embryo.
- ☆ Draw a circle parallel to and above 5mm, above the base of air sac.
- ☆ Using a small corborundum disc cut through the shell at the circle but do not pierce the shell membrane.
- ☆ Apply inchure iodine to the groove cut by the disc and allow drying.
- ☆ Usinf foceps, remove the cap of shell over the air sac to expose the shell membrane.
- ☆ Apply a few drops of sterile saline solution to the shell membrane over the embryo to make the membrane transparent. To cover more than about ¼ of the shell membrane will interfere with the respiration and may result in the death of the embryo.
- ☆ Using a 1ml tuberculin syringe fitted with a 27 gauge, 1 inch needle, insert the needle into the amniotic cavity and inject the inoculums.
- ☆ Close the opening in the shell over the air sac by sealing a disc of sterile heavy paper to the shell with molten wax.

Yolk Sac Inoculation

Procedure

- ☆ Candle 5-7 days old egg and mark the position of embryo and yolk sac.
- ☆ Apply tinchure of iodine ands disinfect the site of inoculation.
- ☆ Drill a small hole through the shell at the upper extremity of the shell over the air sac.
- ☆ Use a 20-22 gauge 1 ¼ to 1 ½ inch needle and insert it perpendicular through the hole to the depth of at least 1 inch and deposit the inoculums.
- ☆ Seal the hole in the egg with molten wax.

Chorioallantoic Membrane (CAM) Inoculation

Procedure

- ☆ Candle 10-12 days old egg and make a pencil mark on the shell below the base of the air sac. Then select a site on the side of embryo about 3mm above and parallel to the base of the air sac for makind the whole without puncturing the CAM.

- ✰ Mark the second site for making hole over the air sac.Apply tincture iodine on both the sites.
- ✰ Make the hole on both the sites taking care not to puncture the CAM with the help of rubber cork containing small pin.
- ✰ For producing an artificial air sac over the CAM, air is sucked with the help of rubber bulb from the hole in air sac. Thus air will pass through the opening made over embryo side permitting the chorioalloantoic membrane to drop from the shell membrane at this point. The embryo membranes and fluid fill normal air sac, thus creating an artificial air sac on the side of egg.
- ✰ Using a 1ml tuberculin syringe with 27 gauge, ½ inch needle, insert the needle through the shell membrane over the artificial air sac and deposit the inoculums on the CAM.
- ✰ Seal the hole with molten wax.

2) Animal Inoculation

The easlist method for virus cultivation which causing human disease was inoculated into human volunteers. In 1900, Reed and Colleagues used human volunteers for their pioneering work on yellow fever. There is serious risk involvement but no other methods available.

In 1909, Landsteiner and popper used monkeys for the isolation of poliovirus but there is high cost and risk to handler's monkeys find only limited application in virology.

In 1903, Theiler used white mice for their work. Mice are still the most widely employed animals in virology.

In laboratory animal (Guinea pig/rabbit *etc.*) may be inoculated by several rout such as intracerebral, subcutaneous, intraperitoneal intranasal.

In virus inoculated animals may be indicated by death, disease or visible lesions. Serial blind passages may sometimes be necessary before evidence of virus growth can be obtained.

Disadvantage

Immunity may interefere withviral growth and that animals often harbor latent viruses. Animal inoculation is also used for the study of pathogenesis, immune response, to test and develop viral vaccines. To raise monoclonal or polyclonal antibodies.

3) Cell Culture

The first application of tissue culture in virology was by Steinhardt and colleagues (1913) who maintained the vaccinia virus in fragments of rabbit cornea.

In 1928, Maitland cultivated the vaccinia virus by using pieces of tissue in nutrient medium.

There is major problem is that bacterial contamination, which can be reduced by adding antibiotics. Since 1949, when Enders, Weller and Robbins reported that poliovirus could be grown in non-neural cells with the production of cytopathic changes. Large numbers of unknown viruses were isolated in cell cultures.

The advantage of cell culture over chicken embryos or experimental animals are.

- ☆ Cell culture can be produced in large quantities and stored at- 70°C.
- ☆ Cell culture gives a clear cytopathic effect.
- ☆ Cell culture can be radiolabile to study the details of virus multiplication.

Three types of tissue cultures are available

a) Organ Culture

In this, small bits of organs can be maintained in vitro for days and weeks. Preserve their original architecture and function. It is usefull for isolation of some viruses. *e.g. Coronavirus.*

b) Explant Culture

Small pieces of tissue can be grown as 'explant' embedded in plasma clots. They may also be cultivated in suspension. This is originally known as 'tissue culture'. Adenoid tissue explants cultures were used for the isolation of *Adenoviruses.*

c) Cell Culture

This is used for routinely cultivation of viruses. Tissues are dissociated into the cells components by the action of proteolytic enzymes such as trypsin and mechanical shaking. The cells are washed, counted and suspended in a growth medium. The growth medium contains essential amino-acids, vitamins, salts, glucose, bicarbonate, 50 per cent calf or fetal calf serum and also added the antibiotics to prevent the bacterial contamination and added phenol red as indicator.Such media will enable most cell types to multiply with a division time of 24 to 48 hours.

The cell suspension is dispensed in milk dilution bottle,tubes *etc.* The cells adhere to the glass surface and on incubation divided to form a monolayer sheet of cells.

Based on their origin, chromosomal charactes and the number of generations through, which they can be maintained, cell cultures are classified into three types.

1. Primary cell culture
2. Diploid cell strains
3. Continuous cell lines

1. Primary Cell Culture

These are normal cells obtained from neonatal or young animals and cultured. They are capable of only limited growth in culture and not maintained in serial dilution. Examples of Primary cell culture are monkey kidney, human embryonic kidney, chcken embryo cell culture. It is useful for isolation and cultivation of vaccinia virus.

2) Diploid Cell Strains

Diploid cell strains are primary cell population that have been sub-cultivated several time, which retain the normal chromosomes constitution of the tissue of origin. After fifty serial passages they undergo 'senescence' diploid strains developed from human fibroblasts are susceptible to a wide range of human viruses. It is useful for isolation of some fastidious pathogens and for production of viral vaccine.

3) Continuous Cell Lines

These are the single types of cancer cells that are the continuous serial cultivation indefinitely. The cell lines is stored at cold (- 70°C) for use when necessary. The established cell lines, their media requirement and virus sensitivity are given in Table 16.1.

Detection of Virus Growth in Cell Cultures

Virus growth in cell culture can be detected by the following methods.

I. Cytopathic Effect

Viruses causes morphological changes in cultured cells. These changes are called cytopathic effect (CPE) and the viruses causing cytopathic effect known as "cytopathogenic viruses".

II. Metabolic Inhibition

In normal cell cultures, the medium turns acid due to cellular metabolism. But when viruses grown in cell culture, there is no acid production due to inhibition of cell metabolism. This can be made out by the color of the phenol red indicator added in the medium.

III. Hemadsorption

In cell culture, when hemagglutinating viruses ie. Influenza and parainfluenza viruses grow, their presence can be noticed by adding the guinea pig erythrocytes to the cultures because when viruses are multiplying in the culture the erythrocytes will adsorbe onto the cell surface. This is called hemadsorption.

IV. Interference

The growth of noncytopathogenic virus in the cell culture can be tested by the subsequent challenge with a known cytopathogenic virus. There first virus growth is inhibited by second virus.

V. Transformation

Oncogenic viruses induce cell transformation and loss of contact inhibition,sothat growth appears in a piled-up fushion producing 'microtumours'.

Table 16.1: Established Cell-lines, their Media Requirement and Virus Sensitivity

Species	*Cell-line*	*Derivation*	*Growth Medium*	*Ratio*	*Morphology*	*Viral Susceptibility*
Cattle	MDBK	Bovine kidney	MEM, 10 per cent FBS	1:10	Fib.	BVD, IBR, VSV
	IMR-31	Buffalo lung	McCoy's 5A, 20 per cent FBS	1:2	Fib.	HSV, BVD, IBR, VSV, Pseudorabies
Hamaster	BHK21/Cl13	Polled kidney from 1 day old Syrian hamster	Eagle's MEM, 10 per cent FBS, 2 mm glutamine, tryptose phosphate broth	1:30	Fib.	EMDV, rabies, Pseudorabies, reovirus, polyoma, VSV, Adenovirus
Human	HeLa	Cervical carcinoma	MEM, 10 per cent FBS, 2 mm glutamine	1:40	Epith.	Poliovirus, Adenovirus
	HEp2	Larynx carcinoma	Eagle's basal medium, 15 per cent FBS, 2 mm glutamine	1:20	Epith.	Poliovirus, Adenovirus
	KB	Oral epidermal carcinoma	MEM, 5 per cent FBS, 2 mm glutamine	1:20	Epith.	Poliovirus, Adenovirus
	Flow-2002	Human embryonic lung	Eagle's basal medium, 10 per cent FBS, 2 mm glutamine, 1 per cent non essential	1:2	Fib.	Poliovirus, HSV, Rhinovirus
Monkey	BSC-1	African green monkey kidney	MEM, 10 per cent FBS, 2 mm glutamine	1:2	Fib.	Poliovirus, VSV, SV40
	Vero	African green monkey kidney	Medium-199, 5 per cent FBS, 2 mm glutamine	1:15	Fib.	Herpes simplex
Mouse	Clone M3	Melanoma cloudman S91	Ham's F 10, 2.5 per cent fbs, 15 per cent horse serum, 3 mm glutamine	1:2	Fib.	Pseudorabies VSV, SV40
	NCTC clone L929	C3H/An mouse areolar and adipose tissue	Ham's F10, 2.5 per cent fbs, 15 per cent horse serum, 3mm glutamine	1:4	Neuroblast	HSV, VSV, vaccinia
	3T3	Swiss mouse embryos	Eagle's medium dulbecco's 10 per cent FBS, 2 mm glutamine	1:20	Fib.	HSV, Polyoma, vaccinia
	3T3	Swiss mouse embryos	Eagle's medium dulbecco's 10 per cent FBS, 2mmglutamine	1:50	Fib.	HSV, VSV, Pseudorabies
Pig	PK15	Clone of pig kidney line PK-29	MEM, 10 per cent FBS, 2 mm glutamine	1:20	Epith.	Hog cholera, FMDV, African swine fever, Vesicular exanthema
Rabbit	RK13	Rabbit kidney	MEM, 10 per cent FBS, 2 mm glutamine	1:15	Epith.	Rubella, Herpes B, HSV, vaccinia

VI. Immunofluorescence

Virus infected cell culture can be stained by fluorescent dye and examined under ultra-violet microscope for the presence of virus antigen. It is widely used for Virological diagnostic purpose.

Infectivity Assay of Virus Preparation

The infectivity of any viral suspension can be measured by making 10 folds serial dilution of virus preparation and inoculating each dilution into a particular host system. *e.g.* Developing chicken embryos or cell culture or even animals to determine the end point of infectivity. The response can be measured in two ways.

I) Quantal response

II) Enumerative response

I) Quantal Response

In Quantal response, the host may die or live or show signs of infection or no infection. The end point is the dilution that kills or infects 50 per cent of assay system used. From this end point and the volume of inocula and its dilution, the titre of the virus can be calculated by applying the formula expressed by Reed and Muench (1938). The titre is expressed as 50 per cent lethal dose (LD_{50}), infective dose (ID_{50}), embryo infective dose (EID_{50}) or tissue culture infective dose ($TCID_{50}$) per unit volume.

II) Enumerative Response/Quantitative Response

The number of lesions on each host. *e.g.* Pock lesion on CAM or plaques in the tissue culture bottle are counted knowing the volume and dilution of virus inoculated, the titre of virus can be calculated as pock forming unit (PFU) or plaque forming unit (PFU) per unit volume.

Fifty Per cent Lethal/Infective Dose

The 50 per cent lethal or infective dose is expressed as doses of viruses that kills 50 per cent of the test animals or infect 50 per cent of chiken embryos/cell monolayers within a given time. As there is variation in the susceptibility of different animals of the same species, the LD_{50} is usually a more practical approach. The LD_{50} or ID_{50} of a particular preparation is usually estimated by reference to the linear mid-section of the dose-response curve in which percentage response between 25 and 75 are plotted against logarithmis of the doses administered. If such an experimental deterimination is not performed with adequate number of animal/assay system, misleading conclusions may be drawn.

Objectives

This is always desirable to know the potency of a virus preparation in terms of its response in a living assay system, which can be determined by ascertaining the mean response to a certain dose and expressed as a unit of measurement. Without the knowledge of potency of a biological preparation, the dose to be given for producing infection or protection against infectous agent in animals can not be calculated. Aslight incrase or decrease in the dose of a virus preparation *e.g.* A vaccinine may lead to absence of protection or immune paralysis.

Methods

- ☆ Make a serial 10 fold dilution of virus preparation in sterile test tube or bijoux using HBSS as diluents.
- ☆ Take 0.9 ml of HBSS in serially arranged test tubes/bijoux and add 0.1 ml virus preparation in the first tube. Mix well and transfer 0.1 ml to second tube and likewise upto the last tube/container.
- ☆ Change the pipette while mixing in each tube/bijoux. All the activities should be done by keeping the containers of the dilution series on ice.
- ☆ Prepare the host for receiving the inocula depending on the assy system to be used.
- ☆ Inoculate 0.1 or 0.2 ml virus preparation from each dilution beginning from highest dilution into 3 or 5 embryos/test tube cultures or Leighton tubes/animals by the specified route.
- ☆ The same syringe can be used to inoculate all the dilutions in a series if the least concentrated suspension is inoculated first. Incubate the assay system at 37°C for desired period
- ☆ The deaths up to 24hours PI are considered non-specific and eliminated from the calculations, after the specified time, record the death/infectivity by the appropriate criteria. The titre of virus is calculated by the method of Reed and Muench (1938).

Example for Estimating 50 per cent End Point

Virus Dilution	*Death Rate*	*Response*		*Cumulative Valve*			*Per cent Mortality*
		Dead ↑	*Alive* ↓	*Dead*	*Alive*	*Ratio*	
10^{-1}	5/5	5	0	24	0	24/24	100.00
10^{-2}	5/5	5	0	19	0	19/19	100.00
10^{-3}	5/5	5	0	14	0	14/14	100.00
10^{-4}	4/5	4	1	9	1	9/10	90.00
10^{-5}	3/5	3	2	5	3	5/8	62.50 x Y
10^{-6}	2/5	2	3	2	6	2/8	25.00
10^{-7}	0/5	0	5	0	11	0/11	0.00

First column indicates dilution of virus used as inoculums

Second column indicates number of embryo/cell culture tubes showing death/CPE over the total number inoculated

Column no.3 and 4 are derived from column no.2

Column no. 5 and 6 are cumulative values obtained from column no.3 and 4 by addition in direction of arrow.

Proportionate distance = Distance X/Distance Y

$$= \frac{\text{Per cent mortality or infectivity above 50 per cent} - \text{50 per cent mortality}}{\text{Per cent mortality or infectivity above 50 per cent - below 50 per cent}}$$

= 62.5 – 50/62.5-25

= 12.5/37.5

= 0.33

Exponential of end point dilution, which produced 50% mortality/infection

= Proportionate distance X difference between exponential of dilution below 50% - above 50% + Exponential of dilution above 50%

= $\{0.33 \times [(-6) - (-5)]\} + (-5)$

= $\{0.33 \times (-1)\} + (-5)$

= $\{0.33 + (-5)$

= 0.33-5

= –5.33

End point dilution = $10^{-5.33}$/unit valve

If the dose inoculated was 0.1 ml, the titre = $10^{-6.33}$/ml

Chapter 17

Genetics of Animal Viruses

Introduction

The virus genetics aims to understanding of the structure and function of viral genome and its products and also study the disease producing capacity and biological properties of the viruses.

Animal viral genetics began with the development of 'Plaque assays' for cytolytic viruses by Dulbecco in 1952.

Genetic analysis of viruses is mutation, which is defined as change or copying of nucleic acid during replication. The change in the gene can alter the viral properties which results phenotypic changes occur in viruses. But not all phenotypic changes that occur with viruses are due to mutation. Mutation could be spontaneous or induced mutations.

The frequency of mutation in viruses is about 10^{-4} to 10^{-8}. In every viral infection mutation occurs. Most mutations are lethal.

1) Spontaneous Mutations

Virus on passage yields a high proportion of mutants in absence of any mutagens. A Thses spontaneous mutation accumulates in the viral genome and produces phenotypic variation. In DNA viruses, There is slow rate of spontaneous mutations is around 10^{-8} to 10^{-11} per incorporated nucleotide whereas RNA viruses exhibit high rate of mutation is around 10^{-3} to 10^{-4} per incorporated nucleotide. The difference in mutation rate between RNA and DNA viruses is due to the differences in the replication enzymes ie lack of proof reading activities in RNA polymerase enzymes.

2) Induced Mutations

Virus mutation can be induced by chemical agents (mutagens like 5-bromouracil and 5- bromodeoxyurudine for DNA virus, alkylating agents and deaminating agents, nitrous acid).

The in-vitro mutagens such as nitrous acid, hydroxylamine or alkylating agents causes chemical modification of the resting nucleic acid cause change in base pairing at subsequent replication and resulting transversions and transitions. The in-vivo mutagens act either by modification of metabolically active nucleic acid or by intercalating the stack of bases. On subsequent replication of the nucleic acid, distorsion of the stack causes the base insertion or deletion.

Types of Mutation

- ☆ Point mutation
- ☆ Mis-sence mutation
- ☆ Non-sence mutation
- ☆ Frameshift mutation
- ☆ Lethal mutation
- ☆ Null mutation
- ☆ Temperature sensitive mutation
- ☆ Plaque morphology mutation
- ☆ Host range mutation
- ☆ Drug resistance mutation
- ☆ Antibody resistance mutation

Point Mutation

Mutation, which occur by single replacement of nucleotide or substitution of one base by another base resulting change in the nucleotide sequence without no change in molecular size is termed as point mutation. This type of mutational changes occurs in higher frequency in single stranded than double stranded nucleic acid. Point mutation can occur spontaneously but its frequency is high if used certain chemical ie. Nitrous acid

Mis-sence Mutation

Point mutation leading to a change in the structure and character of a protein through replacement of amino-acid.

Non-sence Mutation

It is also a point mutation; there is non formation of protein by production of terminal codon.

Frameshift Mutation

In this, multiple insertion and deletions of nucleotide sequences.

Lethal Mutation

Non-production of viable progeny of a test organism.

Null Mutation

In these mutations function of gene is completely inactivated.

Temperature Sensitive Mutation

Lethal mutants are temperature sensitive (ts). The ts mutants have a protein that more easily denatured at higher or lower temperature, active and unable to multiply in susceptible cells at particular temperature. The ts mutants are used for viral genetic studies and development of vaccines.

Plaque Morphology Mutation

These mutants exhibit altered morphology because of metabolic differences in the mutant and the wild type. These mutants are helpful in understanding the egress of virus from the membrane. *e.g. Adenovirus*

Host Range Mutation

These mutants are able to grow on one type of host but not in other.

Drug Resistance Mutation

Drug resistance has been used to assign functions to specific genes or to specific portion of proteins. It is useful control for the specifity of inhibition.

Antibody Resistance Mutation

Such types of mutations have been useful in studies of viral surface proteins, those neutralizing antigens.

Mapping of Mutation

Mutations are mapped by using recombination reassortment methods.

I) Recombination Methods

Recombination between different but closely related viruses and involve in exchange of nucleic acid sequences. It occur more in ds DNA viruses because strand switching by the viral DNA polymerase. This type of recombination also seen in Different types of RNA viruses like as FMD virus and Poliovirus.

Other types of recombination is the reactivation or multiplicity reactivation, which is observed when a cell is infected with two or more viruses of same strain, that have suffered a lethal mutation in different gene and production of infectious progeny. This type of phenomena seen in *Poxviridae, Orthomyxoviridae* and *Reoviridae etc.*

Cross reactivation/marker rescue used to described a different type of genetic recombination between an infectious virus and a related inactivated virus of different genotype with the production of new infectious progeny virus, having genes from both parents. Recombination may take place between the virus genome and host chromosome. No viral progeny is produced but the genetic recombination leads to changes in the host cell such as malignant transformation.

II) Reassortment Methods

There is exchange of complete genome subunits between viruses that have segmented genome. DNA viruses have no segmented genome that's why phenomena confined to RNA viruses like *Reoviruses, Orthomyxovirus, Birnavirus,* and *Bunyavirus and Arenavirus etc.*

There is in-vivo or in-vitro exchange of segments with the production of stable reassortments. This can occur naturally and is important to known the genetic variability among viruses like blue tongue virus.

Chapter 18

Virus – Cell Interaction

When virus replicate on the infected cells. There is cell- virus interaction occurs and also effect on morphological and biochemical alteration that can lead to cell destruction. Some of the viruses are replicate in host cell without producing any detectable effects. Enveloped RNA visuses causes persistant infectinin infected cells.

Large numbers of viruses cause cell damage. Infected cells shows morphological alteration like rounding of cells, cell lysis *etc.* such types of changes reffered to as cytopathic effect (CPE). Several factors play important role in cell death.

a) Partially or complete stop of cellular macro molecular synthesis by viral structural proteins *e.g.* Adenovirus, reovirus.

b) Inhibitory proteins for cellular activity coded by the viral genome. *e.g.* Herpesvirus.

c) Activation and release of lysosomal enzymes into the cytoplasm of infected cells. *e.g.* Adenovirus.

Inclusion bodies – These are the viral specific structures accumulated in the masses in the infected cells. They may be accumulated or situated in the nucleus or cytoplasm or both site. Presence of inclusion bodies in infected cells also give the clue/diagnostic importance that which types of viral infection persist.

Several viruses like *Herpesvirus*, infectious bronchitis virus *etc.* causes fusion of infected cells that leads to syncytia formation. Cell transformation is induced by a number of RNA and DNA viruses, that are characterized by loss of contact inhibition, morphological alteration, reduce growth, chromosomal aberration and antigenic alteration on cell surface.

Interactions between the Viruses Infecting a Cell

When one or more than one virus strain infects a cell. Several type of interaction can take place between such viruses.

1) Non-genetic interactions
2) Genetic interactions

1) Non-Genetic Interactions

a) Complementation
b) Interference
c) Phenotypic mixing
d) Transcapsidation
e) Polylpoid

a) Complementation

When a cells infected by two viruses and if replication titre per cell of either or both of these shows an increase over what it would have been had the cell been infected with either of these, the interaction is termed as complementation. Such interaction is observed when one type of virus is deficient in a particular function that is important for the replication and other virus provides such function. In segmented viral genome, part of the genome gets lost when cells are repeatedly infected with high multiplicity of infection. For certain vital function, such types of virus are unable to grow by themselves and such viruses are called Defective Interfering particles (DI particles). DI particles need supplementation of their deficient function from co-infecting complete virus. Interaction between DI particles and complete viruses is also known as complementation.

b) Interference

When the interaction between two viruses, which leads to drop in titre of one or both of the viruses, phenomena is known as interference.

- ☆ **Heterologus interference** - It can occur between two different viruses
- ☆ **Homologus interference** - It can occur between two related viruses or two strain of same virus.
- ☆ **Autologus interference** – It can occur between virus and DI particles

c) Phenotypic Mixing

Phenotypic charecters may be shared when a cell is co-infected with related viruses, *e.g* influenza virus and paramyxovirus, nucleic acid will be of one parent type and envelops of some progeny virions may contain antigens originating from both parent viruses.

d) Transcapsidation

The genome of one virus and capsid of other viruses, such phenomena called Transcapsidation. *e.g.* retrovirus

e) Polylpoid

When several nucleocapsid are enclosed within an envelop, such type of virion called Polylpoid. All the animal viruses are haploid except retrovirus. Polylpoid can be seen in unmixed infection with paramyxoviruses whereas heteroploid may occur on mixed infections with paramyxoviruses and other enveloped RNA viruses.

2) Genetic Interactions

There is exchange of genetic material is involved. Several types of genetic recombination can takes place, when two different viruses simulataneously infect the same host cell. This recombination may be intramolecular recombination, reassortment and reactivation.

Intramolecular Recombination

Intramolecular recombination take place between different but two closely related viruses during replication nucleiodite sequences are exchanged. *e.g. SV-40* and *Adenovirus.*

Reassortment (Antigenic shift)

Such types of recombination occur in segmented *ss*RNA or *ds*RNA viruses in host cells infected with two related viruses.

Reactivation

Reactivation means activation of non infectious virus by another closely related virus when they are present within a co-infected cell. *e.g. Poxviridae, Orthomyxoviridae etc.*

Cross-reactivation or Marker Rescue

There is activation of infectious and inactivated parent is called cross-reactivation or marker rescue.

Chapter 19

Interferon

Introduction

Issacs and Lindenmann (1957) reported that cell infected with influenza virus contain a non viral substance that could protect cells against infection with the same or a variety of unrelated viruses. This non viral substance was known as interferon.

There are three types of interferons (α, β and γ)

Charecteristics of Interferons

Characters	*IFN- α*	*IFN- β*	*IFN- γ*
Principle source	Leucocyte ds RNA viruses	Fibroblast, Epithelial cells ds RNA viruses	T-lymphocyte mitogen, Antigens
Principle activity	antiviral	antiviral	Immunomodulation
Chromosomal location	9	9	12
Glycoprotein	No	Yes	Yes
Stable at pH 2	Yes	Yes	No
Functional form	Monomer	Dimer	Tetramer

Production of Interferons

The non infected cell (normal cells) does not synthesize interferon due to absence of interferon genes. However interferon is transcribed spontaneously in some cells. All such cell lines are lymphoblastoid cell lines. Some produces IFN – γ but mostly produces IFN- α. The important interferon inducer is virus infection. Both DNA and RNA viruses induce interferon production. In RNA viruses produces better as compare to DNA viruses (except poxvirus). Infected cells produces interferon after4 hours infection and its peak level is when viral protein synthesize and after that declines.

The second type of interferon inducer is ds RNA viruses and replicative form of ssRNA virus and bacteriophages, synthetic ds polyribonucleotides are interferon inducers. The DNA or dsDNA, RNA – DNA hybrid molecules do not induce interferon production.

The third types of interferon inducer are those viruses that are unable to replicate such as viruses in non-permissive cells and inactivated viruses.

Mechanism of Antiviral Action of Interferon

Interferon does not directly in-activated the virus or not directly secreted by infected cells, which destroyed the virus inside it. Interferons react with the cells to depress a second cellular gene. The interferon exerts its antiviral action by the following mechanism:

a) Interferon treated cells produce an enzyme 2^{I}-5^{I} synthetase, which in the presence of ATP and ds RNA synthesizes a group of oligoadenylates collectively called as 2^{I}-5^{I}A. The 2^{I}-5^{I}A in turn activates a specific 2^{I}-5^{I}Adependent cellular endonuclease (RNaseL), which degrade viral RNA and cellular RNA preventing protein synthesis.

b) Interferon treated cells produce protein kinase, which in the presence of ds RNA, blocks initiation of protein synthesis by phosphorylating the protein synthesis initiating factor eIF2.

Inclusion Bodies

Inclusion bodies are intracellular masses that may accumulate either of virions or of unassembled viral components within the infected cells. They may be single or multiple, small or large, round or irregular shape, intracytoplasmic or intranuclear or both, eosinophilic (pink stain) or basophilic (blue stain). These are detected in infected cells by histopathological techniques, immunofluorescence and electron microscopy. *e.g.* Negri bodies in rabies.

Part 4

Chapter 20

Microbiological Staining Techniques

The staining of bacteria and related organisms is one of the important steps in laboratory identification of the disease-producing organisms. The purpose of staining is to render the organisms more clearly visible under the microscope and to differentiate the organisms on the basis of their staining characters. Presence of certain structures in bacteria aid in their identification and different staining methods are also valuable in differentiation of bacteria.

A. Negative Staining

Procedure involves the use of stains for staining of background without staining the bacterial cell. This procedure is useful for study of morphology of the bacteria.

B. Simple Staining

Procedure involves the staining of bacteria with single stain irrespective of characteristics of the bacteria. Commonly used stains include Aqueous methylene blue, dilute carbol fuschin or safranin. Loeffler's alkaline methylene blue is used to show the McFadyean reaction shown by *Bacillus anthracis* and demonstration of metacromatic granules in *Corynebacterium*. McFadyan reaction is a method to demonstrate the capsule. After staining with alkaline methylene blue, the capsule appears pink while the bacterial cell appears blue coloured.

C. Differential Staining

These staining procedures are based on the differences among the different groups of bacterial cells. The procedures, in addition to determining the gross morphology, also serve to differentiate bacteria into two distinctly separate groups.

(a) Gram's Staining

The division of bacteria into two categories indicates a basic chemical difference between two types of cells *i.e.* Gram positive and Gram negative. The research has shown that differences in cell wall composition between two types do exist. A bacterium has a rigid cell wall, which maintains its shape and prevents its disruption under the influence of internal osmotic pressure. This rigidity is due to substance called mucopeptide. The basic differences in two groups are:

1. The **mucopeptide** comprises a major part of the wall substances in Gram +ve organisms, whereas the Gram –ve organisms have relatively little mucopeptide in their cell wall. The cell wall of Gram-negative bacteria is mainly composed of polysaccharides and lipoproteins.
2. The polymer of glycerol and rabitol phosphate known as **teichoic acid** may also be found in the cell walls of Gram +ve organisms but are not present in the cell wall of Gram –ve organisms.
3. The more acidic character of Gram +ve organisms may be responsible for the greater affinity of these organisms for a basic dye.

To explain the Gram's reaction, several explanations have been given. The most reliable explanation is that the gentian violet when applied, enters into the bacterial cells. This is followed by the application of the lugol's iodine. The lugols iodine forms the complex with the crystal violet. The cell wall of the Gram +ive bacteria is impermeable to these complexes and the cells retain them even after decolourization with alcohol. Whereas the cell walls of Gram –ive bacteria is permeable thus allowing escape to the crystal violet-iodine complexes out of the cells. So, after decolourization step the Gram +ive cells remain stained with crystal violet whereas the Gram –ive cells are unstained as the crystal violet comes out under the influence of alcohol. The unstained cells are later stained with safranin to visualize them.

Gram-positive cells become Gram-negative if:

1. Cell is aging (old culture)
2. The cells are mechanically raptured.
3. The magnesium ribonucleotide is removed by the action of enzyme ribonuclease from the protein with which the dye (crystal violet) forms a dye-iodine complex at the surface of the cell membrane.

(b) Acid Fast (Ziehl-Neelsen) Staining

Mycobacteria contain relatively large amounts of lipid material including fatty acids, waxes and complex lipids, of which the mycolic acid is of particular importance. These also contain proteins and a variety of polysaccrides. These organisms have above the average resistance to disinfectants but are destroyed by pasteurization and ordinary heat sterilization. They are resistant to drying and survive for long periods in dried sputum and body fluids.

Acid fast staining is a type of differential staining procedure for bacteria, especially for genus *Mycobacterium*. The Ziehl Neelsen method consist firstly of staining the organisms with a hot, concentrated dye e.i. carbol fuchsin. Heating makes the waxy substances to melt and thereby becomes permeable for dye. Thus dye is allowed entry into the cell. On cooling and rinsing with water, waxy substance gets solidified and seals the pores. Therefore, once stained, the cells resist decolourisation with acid, they are thus 'acid fast'. It is because the permeability of the cells is increased due to application of heat as a result of the melting of the waxy substances (*e.g.* Mycolic acid) and the dye enters into the cells. When the smear cools down, the waxy material again sattles thereby closing the pores. Thus the dye is retained in the cell. In case of non acid-fast organisms, there is no such sealing. Decolourisation is effected with suitable strong acid solution, which allows the draining of the stain out of the cell in case of non-acid fast bacterial cells. The smear is then counterstaind with methylene blue solution. Acid-fast bacteria stain red other bacteria and background stain blue. This method (with 20 per cent sulfuric acid) is used clinically for the detection of *Mycobacterium tuberculosis* in body tissues and fluids (*e.g.* lungs, liver, spleen and urine).

D. Special Staining

(a) Spore Staining

Some of the bacteria form spores under unfavorable conditions. The spores are refractile bodies that are resistant to various physical and chemicals agents. The spores may be spherical or oval in morphology and their position within the cell may be terminal, sub terminal or central. The shape, size and position of spores are the characteristic of the spore forming bacteria and are of importance in identification. Spores are refractory to normal staining procedures and if stained are difficult to decolorize.

(b) Flagella Staining

The motile bacteria posses flagella, which are very thin, thread like appendages present on the cell wall. The length of flagella may be several times more than that of the bacterial cell. The position of the flagella is characteristic and its helps in identification of motile bacteria.

(b) Capsule Staining

Capsule is the outermost layer in the capsulated bacteria. The presence of capsule is considered to be the indication of the virulence of the bacteria as capsulated bacteria are more virulent as compared to non-capsulated bacteria. The capsule is polysaccharide in nature and its thickness is influenced by the medium of growth of bacteria.

(c) Staining of Metachromatic Granules

Method is same as described for Loeffler's alkaline methylene blue staining.

Object: To Study the Bacterial Morphology by Negative Staining

Requirements

Negrosine stain, Bacterial culture, bacteriological loop, slides.

Procedure

1. Mix a loopful of the bacterial culture with equal quantity of negrosine stain on a slide.
2. Spread the mixture on slide with the help of the loop and allow it to dry.
3. Examine under microscope with high power and then in oil immersion objective.

Results

The background appears black and unstained, shinning bacterial cells are clearly visible against dark background.

Object: To Study the Bacterial Morphology by Simple Staining

Requirements

Saturated methylene blue (aqueous) solution/alkaline methylene blue/dilute carbol fuschin or safranin, Bacterial culture, bacteriological loop, and slides.

Procedure

i. Preparation of the smear and fixation

1. Take a clean glass slide and label the slide with a glass making pencil.
2. Sterilize the inoculation loop on the flame.
3. Put a loop full of sterilized distilled water, fresh tap water or saline on the slide.
4. Resterilize the loop and transfer a small portion of the bacterial growth or specimen to be examined onto the drop of water to prepare a light suspension of the material.
5. Spread out the suspension on the slide by holding the loop in a flat position and with oval spiral movements of the loop, move it outwards from the center.
6. Resterilize the loop before setting it aside.
7. Drying: Allow the smear to dry in the air.
8. Fixing: Fix the air-dried smear by passing the slide 3 to 4 times through the flame quickly keeping the smear side upwards. Heat only the bottom of the slide. For capsule demonstration (**McFadyean** reaction) the smear is fixed by dipping in absolute alcohol for 30-60 sec. instead f heat fixation.

ii. Staining

1. Cover the air-dried and fixed smear with the stain and allow it to act for 30 sec. to 1 min.
2. Pour off the stain, wash with water, blot dry and examine under oil immersion objective.

Results

Bacterial cells will appear blue colour.

Object: To Study the Bacterial Morphology by Gram's Staining Method

Requirements

Bacterial culture, 0.5 per cent methyl violet or 0.5 per cent crystal violet, Lugol's iodine, Absolute alcohol, dilute carbol fuchsin, neutral red or safranin.

Procedure

1. Prepare the smear allow it to dry and then fix with gentle heat.
2. Apply crystal violet for 30 sec.
3. Wash with water and apply lugol's iodine for 30-60 sec.
4. Decolorize with absolute alcohol till stain appears to flow.
5. Wash with water.
6. Apply counter stain for 2 min.
7. Rinse with water, bolt dry and see under microscope.

Results

Gram positive	-	Violet
Gram negative	-	Red.

Object: To Study the Bacterial Morphology by Acid Fast (Ziehl-Neelsen) Staining Method

Requirements

Bacterial culture, Carbol fuchsin, Acid alcohol or 15 or 20 per cent sulfuric acid, Methylene blue, slides and sprit lamp.

Procedure

1. Prepare the smear, allow it to dry and then fix with gentle heat.
2. Cover the slide with carbol fuchsin and heat the underside of the slide (with a lighted alcohol soaked swebs or sprit lamp). Stop heating when the slide steams. Keep the slide hot and replenish the stain if necessary, taking care not to allow the smear to become dry. Heat for 5 min, not allowing the staining solution to boil.
3. Wash well with water.
4. Decolorize with acid alcohol or with 1,5 or 20 per cent sulfuric acid. The excess of stain is removed as a brownish solution and the same will become brown. Rinse in water, when the film will appear pink once more. Apply more acid and repeat the rinsing several times until the film appears faintly pink upon washing.
5. Wash well with water.
6. Counter stain with methylene blue for 5 min.
7. Wash well with water and carefully remove the stain deposits from the back of the slide with filter paper.
8. Blot dry and examine under microscope.

Results

Acid fast:	-	Red
Non-acid fast:	-	Blue

Object: To Study the Presence of Bacterial Spore

Requirements

Concentrated cerbol fuchsin stain, Sulfuric acid (0.5 per cent solution), Loeffler's alkaline methylene blue stain, Sporulated culture of bacteria.

Procedure

1. Prepare the smear, air dry and fix over gentle heat.
2. Cover the smear with corbol fuchsin and heat to steam for 3-4 minutes taking care not to boil the stain.
3. Wash with tap water.
4. Decolorize with sulfuric acid (0.5 per cent solution).
5. Wash with tap water.
6. Stain for 2 min with Loeffler's alkaline methylene blue stain.
7. Wash with water, blot dry and examine under oil immersion objective.

Results

The spores stain red while vegetative calls appear blue coloured.

Object: To Study the Presence of Bacterial Flagella

Requirements

Flagella stain, Motile bacterial culture.

Procedure

1. Take 5 ml of an over night broth culture and odd 0.25ml of formalin.
2. Mix and allow to react for 15 min.
3. Add an equal quantity of distilled water, mix and centrifuge at 3000 rpm for 5 min.
4. Decant the supernatant carefully and again add distilled water, mix and centrifuge.
5. Decant as before, resuspend the organisms in 1-2 ml distilled water and make a turbid suspension.
6. Take a perfectly clean slide and flame in blue flame of a Bunsen burner.
7. Draw a line with a wax pencil from the top to the bottom of the slide near the frosted end.
8. Place a 3mm loopful of suspension near the wax line and allow the drop to run the other end of the slide. Allow it to dry.
9. Place the slide on staining rack and add 1 ml of stain warmed to room temperature and allow to act until a metallic sheen is formed on the surface of the stain.
10. Wash the stained slide with tap water without tilting the slide to drain the stain off.
11. Air dry the slide and examine.
12. If required counter stain with 1 per cent Loeffler's methylene blue after washing the flageller stain.

Results

The flagella will appear red colored around blue bacterial cell.

Object: To Demonstrate Presence of Bacterial Capsule

Requirement

Alcoholic gentian violet staining solution, copper sulfate solution (20 per cent), serum, and capsulated bacterial culture.

Procedure

1. Prepare the smear of bacteria in serum air dry and fix by gentle heat.
2. Cover the smear with gentian violet stain and heat up to steaming.
3. Allow the stain to act for 15-20 sec.
4. Wash the smear with 20 per cent copper sulfate solution by several changes.
5. Blot dry and examine under oil immersion objective.

Results

The capsule appears as a faint blue hollow around the dark purple cell body against a faint purple background.

Chapter 21

Demonstration of Fungi

Fungi are morphologically different from bacteria. They are filamentous, gram positive and bear fruiting bodies called spores. Direct microscopic examination by wet mount is probably the most important method of examining and diagnosing mycotic infections in the laboratory. Lectophenol cotton blue staining is specially used to demonstrate the presence of fungi in cultures and tissue specimens and study their morphology.

Object: To Demonstrate Fungi in Skin Scrapings by Direct Microscopic Examination

Requirements

10 per cent Potassium hydroxide solution (KOH), Specimen, Teasing needle.

Procedure

1. Take one drop of 10 per cent KOH solution on a slide.
2. Transfer the specimen (scraping, hair, nails, tissue etc) on to the slide.
3. Tease the specimen with the help of teasing needle to make a thin preparation.
4. Put the cover glass on the material.
5. Leave the slide for 5 min. (or may be long).
6. Alternatively, the specimen may be left in 10 per cent KOH solution for 1 to 2 hrs.
7. Observe under microscope using low power and than high power objectives.

Results

The fungal hyphae and spores will be visible within the digested tissue mass.

Object: To Demonstrate Fungi by Staining with Lactophenol Cotton Blue Stain

Requirements

Lactophenol cotton blue stain, Teasing needle, Specimen.

Procedure

1. Place a drop of stain on a clean slide.
2. Transfer a small amount of specimen in this drop.
3. Tease the specimen if opaque.
4. Place the cover slip on and press down gently.
5. Warm gently to remove air bubbles, if necessary.
6. Examine under low power and then high power objective.

Results

The fungal hyphae and spores will be visible in pale to dark blue colour.

Chapter 22

Demonstration of Bacterial Motility

While most of the specimens for observing presence of bacteria are stained to make them easily visible. The observation of unstained living organisms is required for certain purposes. The bacteria possessing flagella show characteristic motility and this character is used as an identification method for certain specific groups of bacteria. When examining living organisms for the property of motility, it is essential to distinguish true **motility** where by the organisms move in different directions and change their position in the field from either passive drifting of the organisms in the same direction in a conventional current of the fluid or from **Brownian movement** which is an oscillatory movement about a nearly fixed point possessed by all small bodies suspended in fluid and due to irregularities in their bombardment by molecules of water. Motility can be demonstrated by:

Object: To Study Bacterial Motility in Unstained Wet Films

Requirements

Slide, coverslips, live bacterial culture.

Procedure

1. With a glass-marking pen, draw a line across the middle of a slide.
2. Place a drop of culture suspension beside the line.
3. Apply a coverslip to the drop, avoiding trapping of air bubbles.
4. If the film is to be observed for few minutes, seal it against drying by applying nail varnish or molten petroleum jelly to the margins of coverslip.
5. Observe the film with low power lens. Focus the line first and center it in the field. Then focus the line with high power objective. Defocus the condenser by racking it down wards to reduce and diffuse illumination.

Object: To Study Bacterial Motility using hanging Drop Preparation

Requirements

Hanging drop cavity slide, Coverslips, live bacterial culture.

Procedure

1. Take a coverslip and draw a V shaped line on the coverslip with glass marking pencil.
2. Place a small drop of liquid culture or suspension on the same side of coverslip with the angle of V.
3. Take the cavity slide and encircle the concavity with a line steak of soft petroleum jelly applied to the surface of the slide just outside the concavity.
4. Invert the slide over the coverslip, allowing it to adhere to the jelly.
5. Quickly turn round the slide so that the coverslip is uppermost.
6. Proceed to examine first with a low power objective and then with a high power one as described for unstained wet film.

Results

Unstained bacteria are visible in intense, focused illumination. True motility must be differentiated from passive drifting or Brownian movement.

Chapter 23

Determination of Phenol Coefficient

Phenol Coefficient Method

The phenol coefficient of a disinfectant is the highest dilution of the disinfectant divided by hightest dilution of phenol which kills the test organism in 10 minutes but not in 5 minutes under standard conditions.

Phenol coefficient method has been accepted for evaluation of disinfectant. This method is based on principle of tube-dilution method. This test is a specific official test. Phenol coefficient method is also AOAC phenol coefficient method or FDA method.(Association of official agricultural chemists method or Food and Drug aDrug Administration method).

Phenol coefficient method is suitable for testing water soluble disinfectant and exerting their antimicrobial action in a manner similar to that of phenol.

Material Require

Sterile pipettes 5ml, inoculation loop (4 mm diameter) 24 hour old broth culture of Staph.aureus 10 ml, phenol, disinfectant, nutrient broth tubes.

Procedures

- ☆ Prepare a series of dilution of disinfectant and phenol (5 ml in each tube).
- ☆ Phenol = 1/80 1/90 1/100
- ☆ Disinfectant = 1/100 1/150 1/200 1/250 1/300 1/350 1/400
- ☆ Place 10 tubes *i.e.* 3tubes containing 5 ml of different dilution of phenol and 7 tubes containing different dilution of disinfectant in the first row of the rack.
- ☆ Place 10 tubes containing 10 ml broth in each of the second, third and fourth rows of the rack.

- 0.5ml of 24 hours broth culture of the test organism is added in all tubes (Phenol and disinfectant) of Ist row.
- All tubes are incubated in water bath.
- After 30 seconds of inoculation of the last tube of disinfectant, transfer loopful of the material from the Ist tube of the phenol dilution to the first brith tube of IInd row (5 minutes row).
- Continue to transfer one loopful culture from phenol and disinfectant tubes to corresponding brith tubes of 5 minute row.
- After completion of 5 minute row (IInd row) allow 30 seconds to pass.
- Transfer 1 loopful of the material from phenol and test disinfectant dilutions to the corresponding broth tubes of 10 minut row (IIIrd row).
- Transfer 1loopful of the material from phenol and test disinfectant dilutions to the corresponding broth tubes of 15 minute row (IVth row)
- Place the rack in incubator at 37°C for 48 hours and observe the growth.
- Observe the highest dilution of the disinfectant killing the test organisms in 10 minutes but not in 5 minutes.
- Observe the highest dilution of phenol killing the test organism in 10 minutes but not in 5 minutes.
- Calculate the phenol coefficient by

$$\text{Phenol Coefficient} = \frac{\text{Highest dilution of disinfectant that destroys microorganisms in 10 min but not in 5 min}}{\text{Highest dilution of phenol that destroys microorganisms in 10 min but not in 5 min.}}$$

Table 23.1: Media Commonly Used in Diagnostic Bacteriology

Medium	*Uses*	*Sugars and other Substrate*	*pH Indicator*	*Inhibitor*
Nutrient agar	Basic nutritive medium for growth of less fastidious bacteria			
Blood agar	Growth of most bacteria including many of the less fastidious bacteria	Red blood cells (shows haemolysis)		
MC Conkey agar	Growth of Enterobacteriaceae and some other Gram negative bacteria.	Lactose	Neutral red	Bile salts
Brillint grren agar	Salmonella isolation. A few other bacteria will grow on XLD agar	Lactose, Sucrose	Phenol red	Brillent green dye
XLD agar	Salmonella isolation. A few other bacteria will grow on BGA	Xylose, lactose, sucrose, lysine and H_2S detection	Phenol red	Bile salts
TSI agar	Salmonella identification	Lactose, Sucrose, dextrose, and H_2S detection	Phenol red	
Selenite broth	Enrichment broth for isolation of *Salmonellae*			Selenite
EMB agar	Presumptive identification of *Escherichia coli*	Lactose, Sucrose	Eosin and methylene blue	
Edwards medium	Selective for Streptococci; indicates aesculin hydrolysis and haemolysis	Aesculin red blood cells		Crystal violet, thallus sulphate
Purple base agar (1 per cent) maltose	Presumptive differentiation *Staphylococcus aureus* and *S. intermedius*	(1 per cent) maltose	Bromocresol purple	
Chocolate agar	Enriched medium for *Haemophillus* spp.	Lysed red cells X and V factors released		

Table 23.2: Cell Culture Suitable for Isolation of Viruses from Clinical Specimens

Apthovirus (FMD virus)	HEK, HeLa, Hep 2, BHK 21,PK 15, bovine thyroid, IB-RS-2, bovine kidney
Bovine enterovirus	Calf kidney, monkey kidney, pig kidney, BHK 21
Vesicular exanthema	Embryonic tissue culture of pig, horse dog, cat
EEE	CEF, rabbit kidney, Vero, HeLa, rhesus hamster kidney, BHK21,PK 15
WEE	Vero, HeLa, rhesus hamster kidney, BHK21,PK 15
VEE	Chick kidney, Vero, HeLa hamster kidney, BHK21
Japanese encephalitis	Vero, HeLa, CEF, hamster kidney, BHK21, pig kidney cell lines
Bovine virus diarrhea	Bovine kidney, fetal skin, cat kidney, swine kidney
Swine fever (Hog cholera)	Swine kidney, Swine testis, bone marrow, spleen, lymph node, pig kidney
Equine herpes type 1	Primary rabbit kidney
Blue tongue	Bovine and bovine embryonic kidney and testis chang liver, HeLa, BHK21, L929
Vaccinia	RK13, Vero CEF
Herpes simplex 1.2	WI 38,Flow 2002, Vero, FL Amnion
Yaba tumor	BSC 1
Herpes B	RK13, LLC-RK1
Rabbit fibroma, myxoma	Primary canine kidney
Canine herpes	Primary canine kidney
Bovine adenovirus	Primary BEK6, ovine kidney, bovine testies
Human adenovirus	Change conjectiva, HEK, WI38, HeLa, KB, Hep2
SV_{40}	BSC 1, rabbit kidney
Mousepox	Primary MEF
Arenavirus	Vero
Rabbit herpes	Primary rabbit kidney
Vecella zoster	FL amnion, WI38,Flow 2002
Minute mouse virus	MEF
Parainfluenza 3	HEp-2
Srapie	Choroid plexus culture of mouse
Maedi Visna	Choroid plexus culture of sheep
Kuru	Explanted brain cells
Polio	WI38, LLCMK2
Reovirus	Bovine kidney, rabbit kidney, Primary monkey kidney
Retrovirus	Primary CEF
Rubella	RK3
Louping ill	Vero, BHK21, Primary African green monkey kidney
Arican horse sickness	Monkey kidney cell line, BHK21, Vero mosquito cell line

Infectious bursal disease	CEF,CE kidney, Vero
Avian infectious bronchitis	Chich embryo kidney, liver cell, embryonic kidney, Vero
Canine coronavirus	Primary canine kidney
Ranikhet disease	Rabbit, pig, ovine, monkey and hamester kidney and testies, BHK21,Vero, HEK, HeLa, CEF
Canine distemper	Calf, rabbit, hamster, dog and ferret kidney, BHK21,Vero, HEK, HeLa, CEF
Rinderpest	Calf, sheep, goat, hamster, dog and pig kidney and testes, Vero, HeLa, KB, CEF, pig kidney cell line.
Bovine respiratory syncytial	Bovine embryonic and calf kidney, Kidney cell of swine hamster, monkey and man, HeLa, Hep2.
Vesicular stomatitis	CEF, monkey kidney, Vero, HeLa, MEF, BHK21, Pig kidney cell line
Rabies	CEF, MEF, Pig, dog hamster kidney, KB, BHK21, WI 38.
Sheep pox	Kidney and testies of sheep,goat and calf, MDBK
Fowl pox	CEF, Duck embryo fibroblast
Swine pox	Pig kidney and testies, embryo lung and brane culture,PK15
Infectious bonive rhinotracheitis	Bovine, porcine,equine, ovine, caprine, rabbit and human kidney and testies, MFE, CEF, WI38
Pseudorabies	Dog, Rabbit, Pig kidney, Guinea pig testies, CEF, Monkey kidney, HeLa, PK15 bhk21.
Marek's disease	Chick kidney cell, Duck embryo fibroblast
Infectious laryngotracheitis	Chick kidney cell, HeLa
Lymphocytic choriomrngitis	Vero
Malignant catarrhal fever	Sheep thyroid, calf testis, rabbit kidney
Bunya virus	KB,Vero
Corona virus	WI38,Flow 2002
Avian encephalomyelitis	Amniotic cavity of developing chick embryo
Duck virus hepatitis	Amniotic cavity of developing chick embryo
Cytomegalovirus	WI38,Flow 2002
Avian encephalomyeutis	Amniotic cavity of developing chick embryo
Duck virus hepatitis	Amniotic cavity of developing chick embryo
Cytomegalovirus	WI38,Flow 2002
Polyoma	3T2,MEF

Table 23.3: Rapid Diagnostic Tests for Viral Disease of Animals

Viral Disease	*Name of Diagnostic Tests*
Foot and mouth disease	Complement fixation test
Rinderpest	Immunodiffusion, counterimmunoelectrophoresis
Bluetongue	Serum neutralization, immunodiffusion, Immunodiffusion, immunoelectrophoresis
Infectious bovine rhinotracheitis	Immunoelectrophoresis, indirect heamagglutination inhibition
Rabies	Immunoelectrophoresis, immunoenzyme technique, Demostration of negri body by histopathology
Pseudorabies	Immunoelectrophoresis, immunodiffusion
Adenovirus infection	Complement fixation, heamagglutination inhibition
Rotavirus infection	Immunoelectrophoresis, immunodiffusion
Malignant catarrhal fever	Immunoelectrophoresis, immunodiffusion, Serum neutralization
Hog cholera (Swine fever)	immunodiffusion
Mucosal disease	immunodiffusion
Buffalopox	Immunoelectrophoresis, immunodiffusion
Swinepox	Immunoelectrophoresis, immunodiffusion
Sheep pox	Immunoelectrophoresis, immunodiffusion
Goat pox	Immunoelectrophoresis
Marek's disease	Immunoelectrophoresis
Equine herpes virus	Immunoelectrophoresis
Parvovirus	Heamagglunination inhibition
Duck hepatitis	immunodiffusion
Infectious laryngotracheitis	Immunodiffusion
Infectious bronchitis	Immunodiffusion
Avian encephalomyelitis	Immunoelectrophoresis, serum neutralization
Infectious bursal disease	Immunoelectrophoresis, immunodiffusion
Fowl pox	Immunodiffusion
Hepatitis A	Enzymeimmunoassay
Hepatitis B	Enzymeimmunoassay
Influenza	Heamagglunination inhibition
Parainfluenza	Heamagglunination inhibition
Retroviruses	Immunoelectrophoresis, immunodiffusion
Alphavirus	Heamagglunination inhibition
Flavivirus	Heamagglunination inhibition
Swine vesicular disease	Complement fixation test, Serum neutralization
Vesicular stomatitis	Complement fixation test
Vesicular exanthema	Complement fixation test

Table 23.4: Important Viral Diseases of Bovine

Family	*Genera*	*Species*
	DNA Viruses	
Poxviridae	Orthopox virus	Vaccinia virus, Cow pox virus, Buffalopox virus
	Parapox virus	Pseudocow pox virus (milker's nodules)
	Capripox virus	Bovine popular stomatitis virus, Lumpy skin disease virus (Neething virus)
Adenoviridae	Mast adeno virus	Bovine adeno virus type (1 to 8)
Herpesviridae		
Alpha herpes virinae	Bovine herpes virus 1	Infectious bovine rhinotracheitis or infectious bovine postural vaginitis
	Bovine herpes virus 2	Bovine malmillitis virus or pseudolumpy skin disease virus
	Bovine herpes virus 4	Orphan herpes virus
Beta herpes virinae		Bovine cytomegalo virus
Gamma herpes virinae	Bovine herpes virus 3	Malignant catarrhal fever virus
Papovaviridae	Papillomavirus	Bovine papilloma virus (Wart)
	RNA Viruses	
Picornaviridae	Entero virus	Bovine enteroviruses 1 to 7
	Rhino virus	Bovine rhino viruses 1-2
	Apthovirus	Foot and mmouth disease virus-O, A, C, SAT 1-3,Asia 1.
Togaviridae	Pestivirus	Bovine viral diuarrhoea virus (mucosal disease)
Reoviridae	Reovirus	Bovine reovirus type 1 to 3
	Orbivirus	Blue tongue virus type 1 to 24
	Rotavirus	Bovine rotavirus (calf diarrhoeal virus)
Coronaviridae	Coronavirus	Bovine corona virus(calf neonatal diarrhea virus)
Paramyxoviridae	Paramyxovirus	Bovine para influenza 3
	Morbillivirus	Rinderpest
	Pneumovirus	Bovine respiratory syncytial virus
Rhabdoviridae	Vesiculovirus	Vesicular stomatitis virus types 1 and 2, Bovine ephemeral fever virus
Retroviridae		Bovine type-c
Unusual agent		Bovine spongiform encephilitis

Table 23.5: Important Viral Diseases of Equine

Family	*Genera*	*Species*
	DNA Viruses	
Papovaviridae	Papillomavirus	Equine papilloma virus (Wart)
Adenoviridae	Mast adeno virus	Equine adeno virus type (1 to 8)
Herpesviridae	Alpha herpes virinae	Equine herpes virus 1 -3
Poxviridae	Orthopox virus	Equine coital exanthema. Horse poxvirus
	RNA Viruses	
Picornaviridae	Rhino virus	Equine rhino viruses 1-2
Togaviridae	Alphavirus	Equine encephalomyelitis viruses (Estern, Western, Venezualen)
Reoviridae	Reovirus	Equine reovirus type 2 to 3
	Orbivirus	African horse sickness virus type 1 to 9
	Rotavirus	Foal gastroenteritis virus
Orthomyxoviridae	Influenza virus	Equine influenza virus subtype 1 and 2

Table 23.6: Important Viral Diseases of Canine

Family	*Genera*	*Species*
	DNA Viruses	
Parvoviridae	Parvovirus	Canine parvo virus
Papovaviridae	Papillomavirus	Canine oral Papillomavirus
Adenoviridae	Mast adeno virus	Canine adeno virus type 1-2
Herpesviridae		
Alpha herpes virinae		Infectious canine hepatitis virus
	RNA Viruses	
Paramyxoviridae	Paramyxovirus	Canine parainfluenza 2 virus
	Morbillivirus	Canine distemper virus
Rhabdoviridae	Lyssavirus	Rabies virus
Coronaviridae	Coronavirus	Canine corona diarrhea virus

Table 23.7: Important Viral Diseases of Swine

Family	*Genera*	*Species*
	DNA Viruses	
Poxviridae	Orthopox virus	Vaccinia virus
	Suipox virus	Swine pox virus
Adenoviridae	Mast adeno virus	Porcine adeno virus type (1 to 5)
Herpesviridae		
Alpha herpes virinae		Porcine herpesvirus-1 (pseudorabies)
Parvoviridae	Parvo virus	Porcine parvo virus
Unclassified	-	African swine fever virus
	RNA Viruses	
Picornaviridae	Entero virus	Porcine enteroviruses 1 to 9
	Cardio virus	Encephalomyocarditis virus
	Apthovirus	Foot and mouth disease virus
Togaviridae	Pestivirus	Hog cholera virus (Swine fever vius)
Reoviridae	Reovirus	reovirus type 1 to 3
Calciviridae	Calcivirus	Vesicular exanthema virus type 1-13
	Rotavirus	Porcine rotavirus (piglet gastroenteritis virus)
Coronaviridae	Coronavirus	Transmissible gastroenteritis virus
Orthomyxoviridae	Influenza virus	Swine Influenza virus
Rhabdoviridae	Vesiculovirus	Vesicular stomatitis virus
	Lyssa virus	Rabies virus
Retroviridae		Porcine type-c

Table 23.8: Important Viral Diseases of Caprine (Sheep and goat)

Family	*Genera*	*Species*
	DNA Viruses	
Poxviridae	Capripox virus	Sheep pox virus, goat pox virus
	Parapox virus	Lumpy skin disease, Contageous ectyma virus or contagious pustular dermatitis
Adenoviridae	Mast adeno virus	Ovine adeno virus
Herpesviridae		
Alpha herpes virinae		Ovine herpesvirus, Caprine herpes virus
Parvoviridae	Dependovirus	Ovine adeno associated virus
Papovaviridae	Papillomavirus	Ovine and caprine papilloma virus
	RNA Viruses	
Picornaviridae	Entero virus	Ovine enteroviruses
	Aptho virus	Apthovirus (Foot and mouth disease virus)
Flaviviridae	Flavivirus	Louping ill virus
Togaviridae	Pestivirus	Border disease virus (Hairy shaker disease)
Reoviridae	Reovirus	Reovirus type 1
	Orbivirus	Blue tongue virus (Ovine catarrhal fever, sore mouth) types 1-24
	Rotavirus	Ovine rotavirus
Bunyaviridae	Bunyavirus	Narobi sheep disease virus
Lentivirinae	Lentivirus	Maedi-Visna viruses
Rhabdoviridae	Lyssa virus	Rabies virus
Retroviridae		Bovine leukemia

Table 23.9: Important Viral Diseases of Poultry

Family	*Genera*	*Species*
	DNA Viruses	
Poxviridae	Avipox virus	Fowl poxvirus, pigeon pox virus
Parvoviridae	Parvovirus	Goose parvovirus (goose hepatitis virus)
	Dependovirus	Avian AAV, CELO 9Chick embryo lethal orphan)
Adenoviridae	Mast adeno virus	Fowl adeno virus type (1 to 9)
		Inclusion body hepatitis virus, Egg drop syndrome-76
Herpesviridae		
Alpha herpes virinae		Fowl herpes virus-1
Gamma herpes virinae		Avian infection laryngotracheitis, Marek's disease virus
	RNA Viruses	
Picornaviridae	Entero virus	Avian encephalomyelitis virus, Duck hepatitis virus
	Apthovirus	Foot and mmouth disease virus-O, A, C, SAT 1-3,Asia 1.
Flaviviridae	Flavivirus	Louping ill virus
Reoviridae	Reovirus	Avian reovirus type 1 to 5
	Rotavirus	Avian rotavirus
Coronaviridae	Coronavirus	Avian influenza virus (9H 5-6 N subtypes)
Paramyxoviridae	Paramyxovirus	New castle disease virus
Rhabdoviridae	Vesiculovirus	Avian vesiculovirus
Birnaviridae		Infectious bursal disease virus

Glossary

Acid- fast bacteria: Bacteria which are not decolourized by acid alcohol. Acid fastness is an unique characteristics of Mycobacteria.

Aerobes: Bacteria which grow in the presence of environmental oxygen.

Agar: A polysaccharides derivative of sea weed (Algae geledium), used as a solidifying agent in bacteriological media.

Amphitrichous: Flagella at one pole.

Anaerobes: Bacteria which grow in the absence of environmental oxygen

Antibiogram: The antibiotic sensitivity pattern of a bacterial strain.

Antibiotics: Microbial origin substances that kill the bacteria.

Antimicrobial: Antibiotic substances that used against the microbial infection to kill or inhibit the growth of bacteria.

Antiseptic: Substances that prevent the sepsis, putrification or decay by preventing or arrest the growth of microorganisms.

Antitoxin: Antibody produced against microbial toxin and capable of neutralizing the activity of the toxin.

Asepsis: The absence of pathogenic bacteria in living tissues.

Aseptic: Free of microorganisms capable of causing infection.

Atrichous flagella: The bacteria having no flagella.

Autoclave: Instrument used for serilization of liquids, rubber goods *etc.* by moist heat.

Autotrophs: Bacteria got the energy by oxidation of in-organic compounds and carbao dioxide as the sole source of carban.

Axenic: A pure culture of bacterial strain.

Bacillus: Rod shaped bacterium.

Bacteraemia: Bacteria present in the blood.

Bactericidal: Any substances or the mechanism to kill the bacteria.

Bacteriocin: It is a bactericidal agent produced by some of the bacteria that inhibit the growth of other bacteria.

Bacteriophase: Viruses, which infect bacteria.

Bacteriostatic: Substances that inhibit the growth and multiplication of bacteria.

Beta-lactamase: It is a enzymes produced by some of the bacteria that can degrade the penicillin by breakdown he beta lactam ring.

Binary fission: An asexual single nuclear division of bacteria.

Capsule: It is a layer made of sugar that surround the bacterial cell wall.

Chemotaxis: Movements of bacteria from positive to negative direction.

Cocci: Spherical bacteria.

Coccobacilli: An oval shaped bacteria.

Coliphase: Viruse, which infect Eschericha coli.

Colony: Bacterial growth on the solid media that is visible to the naked eyes.

Commensalism: It is a kind of symbiosis in which a bacterium lives at the expense of the host without causing any harm.

Commensals: Bacteria which present in animal body without causing any harm to the animal body.

Conidia: Are the spore of filamentous bacteria produced extracellularly by abstraction from the ends of parent cell.

Conjugation: Is a process of transferring genetic material from one bacterium to other by fusion or with the help of sex-pili.

Culture: The cultivation and growth of microorganisms in suitable medium.

Dipicolinic acid: A compound found in high concentration in bacterial spores.

Diplococci: Cocci occurring oin pairs.

Endemic: Disease present all time in a population abut not always recognizable clinically.

Endogenous bacteria: Bacteria which originates within the host.

Endotoxin: Cell wall of gram negative bacteria made of lipopolysaccharides components that liberate the toxin after breakdown.

Endotoxin: The lipopolysaccharide component of gram negative bacterial cell wall liberated mostly due to disintegration of the bacterial cells and possess toxic activity.

Exotoxin: Toxins or chemical substances excreated by bacteria. Exotoxins are not the integral part of bacterial cell. Most exotoxin are protein and have specific toxic effect.

Facultative anaerobes: Bacteria that grow under in both condition in aerobic or anaerobic condition.

Flagellin: The flagellar protein.

Gene: The functional component of chromosomes that codes for specific polypeptide.

Hanging drop technique: A technique used for determination of motily of bacteria in cavity slide.

Hyaluronidase: An enzyme capable of degrading hyaluronic acid present in the intracellular matrix of connective tissues. It is also called as spreading factor.

ID_{50}: The dose which infect 50 per cent population of experimental animal.

Incubation period: The period of time interval between exposure to infction and the appearance of clinical symptoms of disease.

Infection: A disease state due to the invasion of a host by a pathogenic bacteria.

L-form: A bacteria from devoid of cell wall.

Lophotrichous bacteria: Bacteria having tuft of flagella at one or both poles of the bacterial cell.

Mesophiles: Bacteria which grow best under 20°C to 45°C temperature.

Monotrichous flagella: The bacteria having flagella at one pole.

Obligate aerobes: Bacteria grow only in presence of free oxygen.

Obligate anaerobes: Bacteria grow only in absence of free oxygen.

Pasturization: It is process of heating particularly milk at a controlled temperature and cooling down to destroy the harmful bacteria and enhance the keeping quality.

Peritrichous flagella: Bacteria having flagella all over the surface.

Phototrophs: Bacteria capable of utilizing light energy for metabolism.

Plasmid: Extrachromosomal DNA present in some bacteria. It carries genetic properties and replicate independently.

Pleomorphic: The appearance of bacteria in different morphological forms.

Prokaryote: A cell without true nuclear membrane.

Protoplast: Usually gram positive bacteria with little or no residual cell wall.

Psychrophiles: Bacteria which can grow at low temperature.

Ribosomes: Cytoplasmic structural units made up of RNA and protein and the sites of protein synthesis. Bacteria have 70 S ribosomes each composed of 30 S and 50 S subunits.

Selective media : Media which allows certain bacteria to grow and inhibit the growth of other bacteria.

Septicaemia: A systematic disease condition following the invasion and multiplication of pathogenic bacteria in blood stream.

Sheroplast: Cell wall devoid gram negative bacteria.

Spores: Highly resistant dormant state of bacteria develop under un-favourable condition.

Sterilization: It is process of complete freeing an articles from all forms of microorganisms.

Strain: A pure culture of bacteria.

Symbiosis: It is state in which both host and bacteria benifited.

Thermophiles: Bacteria which can grow at high temperature (50°C).

Titre: The highest dilution of serum that gives positive reaction.

Toxaemia: Presence of toxin in blood.

Toxonomy: The classification of living organisms such as bacteria.

Variant: Bacterium having one or more charecteristics that differ from the parent bacterial strain.

Virulence: It is the degree of pathogenecity.

Highlights

- ☆ The most commonly used endospore stain- **Schaeffer-Fulton stain**
- ☆ Capsule of B. anthracis is made of – **D-glutamic acid**
- ☆ Teichoic acid in Gram-positive bacterial cell wall has- **Glycerol/ribitol**
- ☆ Archaebacterial cell walls usually consists of – **Proteins and polysaccharides**
- ☆ Metachromatin granules serves as a reserve of – **Inorganic phosphate**
- ☆ The chemi-osmotic mechanism of ATP synthesis proposed by- **Peter Mitchell**
- ☆ Reducing media for anaerobic bacteria contains- **Na-Thioglycolate**
- ☆ Mycobacterium leprae is usually isolated in- **Armadillos**
- ☆ Selective media for *S.typhi* is – **Bismuth sulphite agar**
- ☆ Selective media for *Staphylococcus aureus* is- **Mannitol Salt Agar**
- ☆ Paraffin and mineral oils are often sterilized by- **Hot air oven**
- ☆ Sterilizing agent used in space crafts is- **Ethylene oxide**
- ☆ Test used to find the carcinogenicity of mutagens is- **Ames test**
- ☆ Three kingdom classification of bacteria proposed by- **Carl Woere**
- ☆ Pyrogen induced by endotoxins is – **IL-1**

- ☆ Lab test to detect the presence of endotoxins in preparations- **Limulus assay**
- ☆ Resoloving power of a compound microscope is – **0.2nm**
- ☆ Heat resistance of spores is due to presence of – **Dipicolinic acid**
- ☆ Target site of polymyxin is- **Bacterial cell membrane**
- ☆ Thickness of Gram+ve and Gram-ve cell walls are- **20-80nm and 2-7nm respectively**
- ☆ Most abundant membrane protein of Gram-ve bacterial outer membrane- **Braun's lipoprotein**
- ☆ Non-motile asexual sporangiospores of phycomycetes is – **Aplanospores**
- ☆ Exogenously borne sexual spores are known as – **Basidiospores**
- ☆ 'Psuedohyphae is characteristic of – ***Candida albicans***
- ☆ 'North American blastomycosis' is caused by- ***Blastomyces dermatitidis***
- ☆ 'European blastomycosis' is caused by- ***Cryptococcus neoformans***
- ☆ Asexual spores produced by fragmentation of hyphae is – **Arthrospore**
- ☆ Staining used for detection of fungi in pathological specimens- **Periodic acid Schiff stain**
- ☆ Media used for stimulating production of chlamydospores of C. albicans- **Corn meal agar**
- ☆ Method used for observing the development of spores and hyphae of fungus is called- **Block-slide culture technique**
- ☆ Mucor is distinguished from other members of Phycomycetes by- **Absence of rhizoids**
- ☆ Asexual spores of Ascomycetes are known as- Conidiospores • 'Bottle bacillus' is the synonym for- **Pityrosporum ovale**
- ☆ Percent of Agar used for the preparation of solid media is- **1.5 per cent**
- ☆ Microbial population can be maintained in the exponential growth and at constant biomass for extended periods by using- **Chemostat/Turbidostat**
- ☆ The phenomenon by which bacteria monitor their own population density through sensing the level of signal molecules- **Quorum assay**
- ☆ Indicator bacterium used in autoclaving is- ***Bacillus stearothermophilus* (spores)**

- ☆ The commonly used agent for 'cold sterilization is - **Gamma radiation**
- ☆ The disinfectant action of chlorine is due to the formation of- **Hypochlorous acid**
- ☆ Linear chromosomal DNA is found in- ***Borrelia burgdoferi***
- ☆ The topoisomerase that removes the supercoiling during replication- **DNA gyrase**.
- ☆ The negative stain used in electron microscopy is – **Phosphotungstic acid**
- ☆ Bacterium that exhibits directed swimming in response to Earth's magnetic field or to local magnetic fields- **Aquaspirillum**
- ☆ The structure that remain after the treatment of a gram –ve bacteria with lysozyme/penicillin is – **Spheroplast**
- ☆ An inorganic solidifying agent used for autotrophic bacteria- **Silica gel**
- ☆ The procedure for staining the capsular material of B. anthracis is- **MacFadyean reaction**
- ☆ Botulism due to which type of toxin occurs in relation with phosphorous deficiency- **Type D**
- ☆ Vole's Bacillus is the synonym for- ***Mycobacterium murinum***
- ☆ The characteristic 'earthy odour' of the cultures is a feature of- ***Psuedomonas psuedomallei***
- ☆ Swarming growth and fishy odour of colonies is characteristic of- ***Proteus vulgaris***
- ☆ Kauffman-White scheme is used for serotypic differentiation of – **Salmonella**
- ☆ VR (Venkatraman-Ramakrishnan) medium is used as a transport media for - ***Vibrio cholera***

Multiple Choice Questions

1. **Bacteria requiring specific nutrient in the medium for growth is known as:**
   (a) Prototroph (b) Auxotroph
   (c) Wild type (d) None of the above
2. **Time required for sterilization by dry heat is:**
   (a) 160°C for 1 hour (b) 120°C for 3 hours
   (c) 90°C for 3 hours (d) 160°F for 4 hours
3. **Pasteurization process comes under which of the following:**
   (a) Dry heat sterilisation (b) Moist heat sterilization
   (c) Radiation (d) Chemical heat
4. **Vigorously growing anaerobic culture require redox potential is**
   (a) Low (b) High
   (c) Medium (d) Not required
5. **Mycolic acid is present in the cell wall of:**
   (a) Mycobacterium (b) Actinomyces
   (c) Nocardia (d) Corynebacterium
6. **Bacterial cells become smaller during:**
   (a) Lag phase of growth curve (b) Stationary phase of growth curve
   (c) Decline phase of growth curve (d) None of the above

7. **Lympholisation of bacteria is method of which of the following :**
   (a) Freezing (b) Freeze drying
   (c) Chilling (d) Drying

8. ***Mycobacterium tuberculosis* have the generation time in cultures :**
   (a) 20-30 minutes (b) 1-5 Hrs
   (c) 15 Hrs (d) 24 Hrs

9. **Edward Jenner developed which of the following :**
   (a) Small pox vaccine (b) Rabies vaccine
   (c) Foot and mouth disease vaccine (d) Tissue vaccine

10. **Rabies vaccine discovered by :**
    (a) Edward Jenner (b) Louis Pasteur
    (c) Alfred Mayer (d) Debark

11. **The founder of the science of Mycology is:**
    (a) Antony von Leeuwenhock (b) Pier antenio muscheli
    (c) R. Sabouraud (d) Renon and Hueet

12. **Bacteria are :**
    (a) Prokaryotes (b) Lack endocytosis
    (c) Have mesosomes (d) All of the above

13. **Appropriate term for disinfection is:**
    (a) Free of all microorganisms from article, surface or medium
    (b) Destruction of all pathogenic M.O.
    (c) Prevention of infection
    (d) All of the above

14. **Which are not the physical agents used for sterilization :**
    (a) Moist heat (b) Sun light
    (c) Dyes (d) Filtration

15. **Radiation is used in sterilization as:**
    (a) Chemical agent (b) Physical agent
    (c) Biological agent (d) None of them

16. **Natural method of sterilization in water is :**
    (a) Moist heat (b) Sun light
    (c) Dyes (d) Filtration

17. Vigorously growing anaerobic require redox potential:

(a) Low
(b) High
(c) Medium
(d) Not required

18. Which changes does not occur with dry heat in M.O. :

(a) Protein denaturation
(b) Protein coagulation
(c) Oxidative damage
(d) Toxic effect of elevated levels of electrolytes

19. Excellent method for destroying material such as soiled dressing animal carcass:

(a) Hot air oven
(b) Incineration
(c) Moist heat
(d) Radiation

20. Dry heat used for sterilization:

(a) Glassware
(b) Sealpal
(c) Needles
(d) All of above

21. The mesophilic bacteria grow best in temperature:

(a) 0-20°C
(b) 20-30°C
(c) 25-40°C
(d) 40-50°C

22. Psychrophile bacteria grow best in temperature range of:

(a) 0-20°C
(b) 20-30°C
(c) 25-40°C
(d) 40-50°C

23. Which of the following example of psychrophile bacteria :

(a) *Bacillus antracis*
(b) *Pseudomonas aeroginosa*
(c) *Corynebacterium* species
(d) *Actinobacillus* species

24. Which of the following is example of thermophile bacteria :

(a) *Bacillus stearothermophilus*
(b) *Pseudomonas* species
(c) *Vibrio cholera*
(d) All of the above

25. Bacteria living in strictly inorganic environment are called:

(a) Autotroph
(b) Hypotrophs
(c) Barotrophs
(d) None of the above

26. The smallest animal virus known is :

(a) Rabies virus
(b) Rota virus
(c) Blue tongue virus
(d) Foot and mouth disease virus

27. The process of transformation was discovered by :

(a) Griffith
(b) Lederberg and Tatum
(c) Zinder and Lederberg
(d) None of the above

28. The transduction is first studied by :

(a) Griffith
(b) Lederberg and Tatum
(c) Zinder and Lederberg
(d) None of the above

29. The process of conjugation is first of all studied in *E. coli.* by :

(a) Griffith
(b) Lederberg and Tatum
(c) Zinder and Lederberg
(d) None of the above

30. The 'Bacteriophage' is discovered by :

(a) Loeffler and Frosch
(b) Pasteur
(c) Twort and d'Herelle
(d) Ivanosky

31. Examination of wet films or hanging drop indicates :

(a) Shape of bacteria
(b) Shape size of bacteria
(c) Shape, size and arrangement of bacteria
(d) Shape, size, arrangement and motility of bacteria

32. Living cells can be viewed by :

(a) Light microscope
(b) Dark field microscope
(c) Phase contrast microscope
(d) Electron microscope

33. The ultraviolet microscopy was developed by :

(a) Antony van Leewenhock
(b) Barnard
(c) Robert hook
(d) Noll and Ruska

34. Dark field microscope is used for examination of :

(a) Cocci bacteria
(b) Bacillus bacteria
(c) Spirochaetes
(d) Viruses

35. The interference microscopy is used for :

(a) Study of cell organelles
(b) Quantitative measurement of the chemical constituent of cell organelles
(c) Both (a) and (b)
(d) None of the above

36. The resolution power of electron microscope is :

(a) 0.1 nm
(b) 1 nm
(c) 1μ
(d) 10μ

37. The resolution power of electron microscopy is :

(a) 1000 times than the resolution power of light microscope

(b) 10,000 times than the resolution power of light microscope

(c) 100,000 times than the resolution power of light microscope

(d) 100 times than the resolution power of light microscope

38. Type of staining during which the cell is killed :

(a) Vital staining
(b) Intra vital staining
(c) Supra vital staining
(d) None of the above

39. Negative staining is useful for the demonstration of :

(a) Spirochaetes
(b) Bacterial capsule
(c) Both (a) and (b)
(d) None of the above

40. Which of the following is not a differential staining :

(a) Gram's staining
(b) Methylene blue staining
(c) Acid fast staining
(d) All of the above

41. Acid fast staining (current method) was discovered by :

(a) Zeihl Neelson
(b) Erhlich
(c) Both (a) and (b)
(d) None of them

42. Primary stain for the Gram's staining method of bacteria is :

(a) Grams's iodine
(b) Safronin
(c) Crystal violet
(d) None of them

43. Safronin used in Gram's staining act as which of the following :

(a) Primary staining
(b) Counter staining
(c) Mordant
(d) Decolorizer

44. The bacteria which remain purple (violet) color by Gram's staining is called as :

(a) Gram positive
(b) Gram negative
(c) Both (a) and (b)
(d) None of them

45. Which are acid fast bacteria :

(a) Gram positive
(b) Gram negative
(c) Both (a) and (b)
(d) Gram variable bacteria

46. Acid fastness of mycobacteria species is due to :

(a) High molecular weight of cell wall content
(b) Mycolic acid
(c) Both combinedly responsible
(d) None of the above

47. Bacteria which remain red colored after Zn staining are :

(a) Acid fast bacteria
(b) Partial acid fast bacteria
(c) Non acid fast bacteria
(d) Gram variable bacteria

48. Which of the following is the uniform rod shaped bacteria :

(a) *Corynaebacteria*
(b) *Bacillus anthracis*
(c) *Mycobacteria*
(d) *Streptococci*

49. Which of the following are branching filamentous bacteria :

(a) *Bacillus anthracis*
(b) *Actinomyces*
(c) *Actinobacillus*
(d) *Mycobacteria*

50. Which of the following is the example of cocobacillia :

(a) *Pasteurella* species
(b) *Yersinia* species
(c) *Haemophilus* species
(d) All of the above

51. Which is the cell wall less bacteria :

(a) Rickettsia
(b) Chlamydia
(c) Mycoplasma
(d) Spirochaetes

52. Which layer of cell envelope is responsible for characteristic shape of bacteria

(a) Cell membrane
(b) Cell wall
(c) Protoplasm
(d) All of the above

53. Techoic acid is present in the cell wall of :

(a) Gram positive
(b) Gram negative
(c) Both (a) and (b)
(d) None of them

54. Lipopolysaccharide (LPS) is present in the cell wall of which bacteria :

(a) Gram positive
(b) Gram negative
(c) Both (a) and (b)
(d) None of them

55. Cell envelope of bacteria consist of layers in which order from inside to outside :

(a) Plasma membrane, Outer membrane, Peptidoglycon layer
(b) Plasma membrane, Peptidoglycon layer, Outer membrane
(c) Peptidoglycon layer, Plasma membrane, Outer membrane
(d) Outer membrane, Peptidoglycon layer, Plasma membrane

56. LPS of gram negative bacteria is responsible for :

(a) Endotoxic activity
(b) 'O' Antigenic specificity
(c) Both (a) and (b)
(d) None of the above

57. Gram positive bacteria consisting cytoplasmic membrane and its contents is called as :

(a) Spheroplast (b) Bacteria ghost

(c) Protoplast (d) None of them

58. Bacterial cell have which ribosomes :

(a) 70s (b) 60s

(c) 80s (d) 40s

59. Deoxyribonucleioprotien found in which of the following :

(a) Prokaryotic cells (b) Eukaryotic cells

(c) Both (a) and (b) (d) None of them

60. Extra nuclear circular self replicating DNA of the bacteria is called as :

(a) Chromosome (b) Episome

(c) Ribosome (d) Centrosome

61. Capsule of bacteria is generally made up of :

(a) Polypeptides

(b) Polysaccharides

(c) Lipids

(d) Mixture of the protein and carbohydrates

62. Capsule can easily demonstrated by which of the following :

(a) Methylene blue (b) Giemsa stain

(c) Acid faststain (d) India ink

63. Bacterial flagella is made up of :

(a) Pillin protein (b) Flagellin protein

(c) Gelatin protein (d) Core protein

64. Flagella in *Salmonella typhii* have the pattern of :

(a) Lophotrichous (b) Peritrichous

(c) Monotrichous (d) Amphitrichous

65. Locomotory organ of spirochaeta bacteria are :

(a) Flagella (b) Pilli

(c) Axial filaments (d) Prendopodia

66. Pilli or fimbrae are found in which of the following :

(a) Gram positive bacteria (b) Gram negative bacteria

(c) Both (a) and (b) (d) Fungi

67. Calcium dipicolinic acid is found in which state of bacterial cell :

(a) Vegetative state (b) Spore coat

(c) Reproduction state (d) Dividing state

68. Maximum growth rate of a bacterium is dependent upon :

(a) Genetic makeup (b) Environment

(c) Nutrition (d) None of the above

69. Lag phase in the bacterial growth refers to :

(a) Adaptation to the old environment

(b) Adaptation to the new environment

(c) Dormancy

(d) None of the above

70. Pathogenic bacteria most commomly grow optimally at pH :

(a) pH 6 - 7.4 (b) pH 7.2 -7.4

(c) pH 7.4 - 8.6 (d) pH 8.2 – 10.0

71. Most of the pathogen of warm blooded animals are :

(a) Thermophiles (b) Mesophiles

(c) Psychrophiles (d) None of them

72. The cell of bacteria is made up of :

(a) Glycolipids (b) Glycoproteins

(c) Lipoproteins (d) Micropeptides

Fill in the Blanks

1. Koch's postulates was derived by using which bacterium ________ ?
2. Father of Microbiology ________
3. Father of Bacteriology ________
4. Small pox vaccine was developed by ________ in the year1796.
5. A polymer of glycerol phosphate that is present only in G+ bacteria cell wall ________
6. Rabies vaccine was first done on ________
7. Loeffler and Frosch shares the credit of discovery of ________
8. The only anti TB drug that has the ability to destroy the acid fastness of Mycobacterium ________

9. The bacteria that is used to evaluate the phenol coefficient using Rideal Walker method _______
10. The substance present normally in spores at high levels, but decreases during the favourable condition _______
11. In Mc Konkeys agar, *E.coli* produces _______ colonies whereas Salmonella produces _______
12. Ringer and Gillespie medium is used for the growth of _______
13. In H and E staining T.B. calcification appear as _______ colour.
14. Two medium used for the growth of mycoplasma _______ / _______

Answers Key

Multiple Choice Questions Key

1	(b)	2	(a)	3	(b)	4	(a)
5	(a)	6	(a)	7	(b)	8	(d)
9	(a)	10	(b)	11	(a)	12	(d)
13	(b)	14	(c)	15	(b)	16	(b)
17	(a)	18	(b)	19	(b)	20	(d)
21	(c)	22	(a)	23	(b)	24	(a)
25	(a)	26	(d)	27	(a)	28	(c)
29	(b)	30	(c)	31	(d)	32	(a)
33	(b)	34	(c)	35	(c)	36	(a)
37	(c)	38	(c)	39	(c)	40	(b)
41	(a)	42	(c)	43	(b)	44	(a)
45	(a)	46	(c)	47	(a)	48	(a)
49	(b)	50	(d)	51	(c)	52	(b)
53	(a)	54	(b)	55	(b)	56	(c)
57	(c)	58	(a)	59	(b)	60	(b)
61	(b)	62	(d)	63	(b)	64	(b)
65	(a)	66	(b)	67	(d)	68	(c)
69	(b)	70	(b)	71	(b)	72	(d)

A) Fill in the Blank

1. *Bacillus anthracis*
2. Louis Pasteur
3. Robert Koch
4. Edward Jenner
5. Teichoic acid
6. Joseph Meister
7. FMD Virus
8. Izoniazid
9. *Salmonella typhi*
10. Calcium Dipicolinate
11. Pink; Colourless
12. Leptospira
13. Blue
14. PPLO Agar and Frey's medium

Appendix

A) Staining Solutions

Negative Staining

Water soluble Negrosin	10 g
Distilled water (D.W.)	100 ml

Immerse the stain in boiling water for 30 min. and then add 0.5 ml formalin. Filter through filter paper before use.

Aqueous Methylene Blue

Saturated solution of Methylene blue (1.5 per cent)	5 ml
D.W.	95 ml

Mix thoroughly and filter before use.

Loeffler's Alkaline Methylene Blue

Soln- A Methylene blue	0.3
Ethyl alcohol (95 per cent)	30.0 ml

Soln- B Dilute potassium hydroxide (0.01 per cent) 100 ml

Mix solution A and B to prepare the staining solution.

Gram's Staining

(a) Hacker's Crystal Violet

Soln- A	Crystal violet powder	2 g
	Ethyl alcohol	20 ml

Soln- B	Ammonium Oxalate	0.8 g
	D.W.	80 ml

Mix Soln A and B store for 24 h and filter through coarse filter paper.

(b) Gram's Iodine

Iodine	10 g
Potassium Iodide	2.0 g
D.W.	300 ml

Dissolve the ingredients using pestle and mortar and filter.

(c) Hacker's Counter Stain

Safranin O	2.5 g
Ethyl alcohol	100 ml

For use add 10 ml of stock soln to 90 ml of D.W.

Acid Fast Staining

(a) Carbol Fuchsin

Soln- A Basic Fuchsin	3.0 g
Soln- B Liquefied phenol	5.0 ml
D.W.	95 ml

Mix 10 ml of Soln A with 90 ml of Soln B.

(b) Acid Alcohol Soln

Ethyl alcohol (95 per cent)	5.0 ml
Hydrochloric acid (conc.)	95 ml

(c) Counter Stain

Methylene Blue	0.3 g
D. W.	100 ml

Capsule Stain

Soln- A	Saturated alcoholic solution of gention violet 5ml	
	D. W.	95 ml
Soln- B	Copper sulphate	20 g
	D.W.	100 ml

Dissolve copper sulphate cryslats in the D.W. by gentle heating and filter

Flageler Stain

Soln- A	Basic Fuchisn	0.6 g
	Ethyl alcohol	50 ml

Shake and let stand over night to dissolve

Soln-B	Tannic Acid	1.5 g
	Sodium chloride	0.75 g
	D. W.	100 ml

Mix solution A and B thoroughly.

Lacto Phenol Cotton Blue Stain

Lactic Acid	20 g
Phenol crystals	20 g
Glycerin	40 g
D.W.	20 ml

Dissolve the ingredient by heating gently over the steam bath

To prepare the stain add 0.05 g of cotton blue dye to the above solution. Mix thoroughly and Filter before use.

Tetrathionate Vroth

Calcium carbonate, $CaCO_3$	2.5g
Nutrient broth	78 ml
Thiosulphate solution	15 ml
Iodine solution	4 ml
Phenol red, 0.02 per cent in 20 per cent ethanol	3 ml

Peptone Water for Sugar Fermentation Test

Peptone	1.0 g
Sodium chloride	0.5 g
Distilled water	100 cc
Sugar	1.0 per cent
pH	7.4 – 7.5

Lab Lamco Media

Lab lamco	20 g
Eupeptone	20 g
Sodium chloride	10 g
Distilled water	1,000 ml

Index

C

D

E

M

N

O

P

www.ingramcontent.com/pod-product-compliance
Ingram Content Group UK Ltd.
Pitfield, Milton Keynes, MK11 3LW, UK
UKHW020814290926
15470UKWH00003B/1157

9 789387 057326